Aging and Chronic Disorders

Stephen J. Morewitz   Mark L. Goldstein

Aging and Chronic Disorders

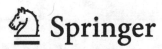
Springer

Stephen J. Morewitz, PhD
Stephen J. Morewitz, PhD &
  Associates
Buffalo Grove, IL 60089
USA
morewitz@earthlink.net

Mark L. Goldstein, PhD
Northbrook, IL 60062
USA
mlgLmr@aol.com

ISBN-13: 978-1-4419-4362-0   e-ISBN-13: 978-0-387-70857-7

Printed on acid-free paper.

9 8 7 6 5 4 3 2 1

springer.com

This book is dedicated to Dad and Lora, Sharone, Lisa, Ashley, and Jonathan

Preface

Five of the six leading causes of death among older Americans in 2004 were chronic diseases, such as cardiovascular disease, cancer, cerebrovascular disease (stroke), chronic pulmonary disease, and diabetes mellitus. All of these diseases negatively affect quality of life, contributing to reduced functioning and the increased eventuality of having to move to a nursing home or retirement community. The increased birth rate after World War II and the significant increase in life expectancy since the early twentieth century have resulted in an increased prevalence of disabling and costly chronic diseases.

There are many questions still to be addressed in the fields of aging and chronic disease. What are the risk factors associated with the increased prevalence of chronic diseases in older populations? What are the major complications that contribute to disability and increased health care utilization and costs? What impact do chronic diseases have on disability and quality of life? What are the most effective treatments and rehabilitation programs? What steps can be taken to avoid overuse and/or misuse of drugs? How can patient education and self-management activities be improved to help these patients and their caregivers better understand and cope with their conditions? How can caregiver burden be reduced?

This book addresses these questions by focusing on how major chronic disorders, such as diabetes, arthritis, cardiovascular disease, and cancer, affect health care utilization, costs, coping, disability, and quality of life in aging populations. Research studies are used to illustrate a wide range of topics from the epidemiology of chronic diseases in older populations, health care utilization and costs, to quality of life concerns, treatment outcomes, and caregiver burden. Case studies from a clinical psychologist's private practice are used to clarify some psychosocial issues underlying chronic diseases and health care.

Chapter 1 analyzes the epidemiology of eight chronic diseases in older adults. Data on the prevalence of diseases and associated risk factors are stressed in this chapter. Health care planners can use these analyses to improve primary and secondary health care prevention activities through more effective uses of health care resources.

Chapter 2 examines the latest information on health care utilization and costs for older adults that can point to a more efficient means of reducing the rising health care costs associated with the treatment of chronic diseases.

In Chaps. 3-5, Dr. Mark L. Goldstein, a clinical psychologist, reviews the literature and uses composite case studies from his practice to illustrate quality of life issues, psychosocial problems, and cognitive difficulties in older adults.

In the remaining chapters, each of the eight chronic diseases is evaluated in terms of five major issues. First, the latest trends in complications associated with each chronic condition are explored. Second, the impact of each disease on disability and quality of life is analyzed. Third, the processes of stress, coping, and social support are described. Fourth, the latest information on treatment and rehabilitation outcomes is discussed. Last, new trends in patient education and self-management are presented.

The information in this book will be relevant to a wide range of professionals and students in the fields of gerontology, medicine, nursing, public health, mental health, social work, education, health administration, health policy, and social sciences.

Buffalo Grove, Illinois   Stephen J. Morewitz
Northbrook, Illinois   Mark L. Goldstein

Acknowledgments

I would like to thank Mrs. Myra Kalkin Morewitz and Dr. Harry A. Morewitz for their advice and support. I also want to thank Bill Tucker, Executive Editor, Health and Behavior, at Springer, who has been supportive as well as thorough and thoughtful.

Buffalo Grove, Illinois   Stephen J. Morewitz
Northbrook, Illinois   Mark L. Goldstein

List of Abbreviations and Acronyms

ACE—angiotensin-converting enzyme
AD—Alzheimer's disease
ADLs—activities of daily living
AF—atrial fibrillation
AIDES—Assessment, Individualization, Documentation, Education, Supervision
ALOS—average length of stay
AMI—acute myocardial infarction
BMD—bone mineral density
BP—back pain
CAD—coronary artery disease
CAM—complementary and alternative medicines
CDC—Centers for Disease Control and Prevention
CGA—comprehensive geriatric assessment
CHD—coronary heart disease
CHF—congestive heart failure
CLBP—chronic low back pain
CR—cardiac rehabilitation
CT—computerized tomography
DM—diabetes mellitus
DMARD—disease modifying anti-rheumatic drugs
EEG—electroencephalogram

EPESE—Established Population for the Epidemiological Study of the Elderly
EPIC—European Prospective Investigation of Cancer
ESRD—end-stage renal disease
FDA—Food and Drug Administration
FFS—fee-for-service
FM–fibromylgia
HABC—Health, Aging and Body Composition Study
HEARTFELT—Heart Failure Effectiveness & Leadership
HF—heart failure
HMO—health maintenance organizations
HRQL—health-related quality of life
IA—inflammatory arthritis
IADLs—instrumental activities of daily living
IVR—Interactive Voice Response
LAC—laparoscopic assisted colectomy
LBP—low back pain
LED—lower extremity disease
LPN—licensed practical nurse
MC—managed care

MI—myocardial infarction
MMN—mismatch negativity
MMWR—Morbidity & Mortality Weekly Report
MRIs—magnetic resonance imaging
MS—multiple sclerosis
NA—nursing assistant
NCHS—National Center for Health Statistics
NHANES—National Health and Nutrition Examination Survey
NIH—National Institutes of Health
NSAIDS—non-steroidal anti-inflammatory drugs
NSCLC—non-small-cell lung cancer
OA—osteoarthritis
OP—osteoporosis
OTC—over-the-counter
PAD—peripheral arterial disease
PAID—Problem Areas in Diabetes Protocol
PENS—percutaneous electrical nerve stimulation
PET—positron emission tomography
PM—particulate matter
PPO—preferred provider organizations

PSA—prostate-specific antigen
PTH—parathyroid hormone
PTSD—post traumatic stress disorder
QSD-R—Questionnaire on Stress in Patients with DM
RA—rheumatoid arthritis
REM—rapid eye movement
SCLC—small-cell lung cancer
SES—socioeconomic status
SF-36—Short-Form-36 Health Survey
SHAPE—Screening for Heart Attack Prevention and Education
SLUMD—St. Louis Mental Status Exam
STEMI—ST elevation myocardial infarction
TEMS—transanal endoscopic microsurgery
TM—transcendental meditation
TME—total mesorectal excision
TNF—tumor necrosis factor
UFT-tegafur/uracil
USDHHS—U.S. Department of Health and Human Services
VA—Department of Veterans Affairs
VATS—video-assisted thoracoscopic resection

Contents

1
Chronic Disorders in an Aging Population: Epidemiology

Life expectancy in the U.S. has risen consistently since the early Twentieth century. In 1900, life expectancy at birth was 47.3 years and in 2004 it was a record high of 77.9 years (NCHS E Stats, 2004; Shi and Singh, 2004). In addition, the birth rate increased after World War II, resulting in the baby boom generation. As a result, the U.S. is having an increase in the elderly population. Between 2000 and 2030, the proportion of the U.S. population 65 years and over is projected to rise from 12.4% to 20%, or one in five, between 2000 and 2030.

With the aging boom, there is, and will continue to be an increased prevalence of chronic diseases in older adults, such as cardiovascular disease, cancer, cerebrovascular disease, chronic pulmonary disease, and diabetes mellitus (DM) (Morewitz, 2006). An investigation of Medicare recipients showed that 82% suffered from at least one chronic disease, and 65% suffered from multiple diseases (Wolff, et al., 2002). In 2001, the leading causes of death among people aged 65 and over were heart disease, cancer, cerebrovascular diseases (stroke), chronic respiratory diseases, influenza and pneumonia, and DM (Federal Interagency Forum on Aging-Related Statistics, 2004).

The prevalence of chronic conditions varies by gender (Federal Interagency Forum on Aging-Related Statistics, 2004). Women have a higher prevalence of hypertension, asthma, chronic bronchitis, and arthritic symptoms than men. Men report higher levels of cancer, DM, and emphysema than women. Men also have higher levels of cardiovascular disease than women. However, by age 75, cardiovascular disease is more prevalent among women than men (Elhendy, et al., 2006).

There are ethnic and racial differences in the prevalence of certain chronic diseases (Federal Interagency Forum on Aging-Related Statistics, 2004). Among people, aged 65 years and over, non-Hispanic blacks have a higher prevalence of hypertension and DM than non-Hispanic whites (66% vs. 49% for hypertension and 23% vs. 14% for DM). Hispanics also have a higher prevalence of DM than non-Hispanic whites (24% vs. 14%) but have a similar prevalence of hypertension (48%).

The prevalence of some conditions is increasing over time (Federal Interagency Forum on Aging-Related Statistics, 2004). Forty-seven percent of people, aged 65 years and over, reported having hypertension in 1997-1998, compared with 50% in 2001-2002. Likewise, DM is increasing among older adults, from 13% in 1997-1998 to 16% in 2001-2002.

Older adults with chronic diseases face substantial disability. More than one-third on non-institutionalized adults, aged 65 years and older, had impairment in activities in 2003 (USDHHS, Health, United States, 2005). The percent of seniors, aged 85 years and older, having a limitation in activities was more than twice that of seniors in the 65 to 74 year age group. For seniors, arthritis and musculoskeletal conditions were the most frequently reported conditions that produced any impairment in activities. The second was cardiovascular disease and other circulatory problems, including stroke. For adults, aged 85 years and older, senility (including Alzheimer's disease and other forms of dementia), poor vision, and hearing loss were the most commonly reported causes of limitation in activities.

In terms of specific types of impairments, 3% of seniors, aged 65 to 74 years, in 2003 reported having limitations in their basic activities of daily living (ADLs), e.g., eating, bathing, dressing, and moving around the house (USDHHS, Health, United States, 2005). Ten percent of seniors, aged 75 years and older, reported having impairments in ADLs. More than 90% of institutionalized Medicare beneficiaries had impairments in ADLs.

In 2003, 12% of non-institutionalized seniors reported impairment in instrumental activities of daily living (IADLs), e.g., managing money, shopping, performing housework (USDHHS, Health, United States, 2005). As in the case of ADLS, impairment in IADLs increase with age. Seven percent of adults in the 65 to 74 age group reported limitations in IADLs, while 18% of seniors, aged 75 and older, reported IADLs impairments.

Below is more detailed information on the epidemiology of eight chronic conditions that afflict persons 65 years and older.

Diabetes (DM)

The prevalence of diabetes mellitus (DM) is increasing around the world. An estimated 30 million persons had DM in 1985, and the number had increased to more than 150 million in 2000 (International Diabetes Federation, 2006). By 2025, the number of individuals with DM is projected to increase to almost 350 million.

DM is most prevalent among older adults in many populations (International Diabetes Federation, 2006). A study of Medicare beneficiaries, aged 67 years and older, revealed that the annual rate of newly diagnosed DM increased by 36.9% between 1994 and 2001 (McBean, et al., 2004). However, the prevalence of DM is also increasing among younger age groups.

In developed countries, the prevalence of DM is higher than in developing countries (International Diabetes Federation, 2006). However, it is projected that in the future, developing countries will have the highest rates of increase in the disease. Several factors, such as increased urbanization, westernization, and economic development in developing countries influence the increase in the prevalence of DM (International Diabetes Federation, 2006). Traditional lifestyles and nutritional patterns are disappearing with the spread of urbanization, industrialization, westernization and economic development. The rapid increase in the prevalence of DM in the U.S. and around the world is due to the aging of the population, consumption of unhealthy food, overweight and obesity, and a sedentary lifestyle (International Diabetes Federation, 2006). These tends are likely to continue.

The number of persons in the U.S. with DM more than doubled from 5.8 million to 14.7 million between 1980 and 2004 (Centers for Disease Control and Prevention, Data & Trends). About 5.1% of Americans reported that they had DM. Persons, aged 65 years or older, make up almost 40% of the people with DM. In 2004, persons aged 65 to 74 years, (16.7%) had about 12 times higher prevalence of diagnosed DM than persons younger than age 45 years (1.4%).

The age-adjusted prevalence of diagnosed DM for men and women was similar between 1980 and 1998 (Centers for Disease Control and Prevention, Data & Trends). However, in 1999, the DM rate for males started to overtake and surpass that of females. By 2004, the age-adjusted prevalence of diagnosed DM went up to 81% for males and 59% for females.

In 2004, the prevalence of diagnosed DM was higher for African-Americans and Hispanics than for whites for persons of all age groups (Centers for Disease Control and Prevention, Data & Trends). The prevalence tended to be highest among individuals aged 65 years or older and lowest among those younger than 45 years of age, regardless of gender and race/ethnicity.

According to "Centers for Disease Control and Prevention, Data & Trends", the self-reported prevalence of any cardiovascular disease in 2003 was higher among those aged 75 years or older (58%) and aged 65 to 74 years (48%) than among those aged 35 to 64 years (27.8%).

Arthritis

In the U.S., about 46 million persons, or 1 in 5, are afflicted with some form of arthritis, making it one of the most prevalent chronic disorders (CDC, National Center for Chronic Disease Prevention and Health Promotion, 2003-2005). More than 38% or 17 million adults with arthritis are impaired in their functioning because of their diseases. By 2030, the number is expected to be nearly 67 million or 25% of U.S. adults due in large part to the aging of the U.S. population. Those with impairments related to arthritis are projected to increase from 16.9 million (7.9%) to 25 million (9.3% of U.S. adults).

One of every two individuals over the age of 65 is affected by arthritis. The prevalence rates are higher for women, older people, those in rural areas, and those with low socioeconomic status (About Arthritis). Genetic factors, obesity, joint injuries, infections, and labor-intensive occupations also increase the risk of arthritis.

Whites and African-Americans have similar prevalence rates (15% and 15.5%, respectively), while Hispanics and Asian/Pacific Islanders have lower rates (11.3% and 7.3%, respectively) (About Arthritis). By 2020, it is expected that arthritis will afflict 49.7 million whites, 7 million African-Americans, 5.1 million Hispanics, 1.6 million Asians/Pacific Islanders, and 442,000 Native Americans/Alaskan Natives. It is projected that by 2020, arthritis will limit the activity of about 9.3 million whites, 1.8 million African-Americans, 1.2 million Hispanics, 264,000 Asian/Pacific Islanders, and 115,000 Native Americans and Alaskan Natives (MMWR Weekly, 1996).

Osteoarthritis (OA)

Osteoarthritis (OA) is the most prevalent type of arthritis, afflicting 12.1% of U.S. adults or 20.7 million individuals (NIH News Release, 1998). OA, also known as degenerative joint disease, is the second to chronic heart disease as the most common diagnosis.

Rheumatoid Arthritis (RA)

Rheumatoid arthritis (RA) is an autoimmune disease that produces inflammation with pain, stiffness, swelling, and deformity in the joints (NIH News Release, 1998). RA can also influence connective tissue and blood vessels in the body, causing inflammation in various organs, including the lungs and heart, and can increase an individual's risk of dying from respiratory and infectious diseases (National Arthritis Plan, 1999). The disease afflicts about 1% of adults in the U.S., most of who are women. About 1.5 million women and 600,000 men are affected (NIH News Release, 1998).

Osteoporosis (OP)

Osteoporosis (OP) is a prevalent, preventable skeletal disease that consists of bone loss and decreased bone quality, thus making its victims predisposed to fractures typically of the hip, spine, and wrist (American Association of Orthopaedic Surgeons, 1999; Wilkins and Birge, 2005). OP is considered a polygenic disorder that is influenced by different genes and environmental factors (Andrew and Macgregor, 2004).

OP afflicts more than 200 million individuals around the world (American Association of Orthopaedic Surgeons, 1999). In the U.S., 10 million persons have OP and 18 million are at risk for the disease. In the U.S., OP is highest among women, non-blacks, and individuals 70 years and older (U.S. Department of Health & Human Services-Public Health Service, 2002). Caucasian and Asian women have a higher incidence of OP fractures than African-American and Hispanic women (American Association of Orthopaedic Surgeons, 1999). However, the risks for African-American and Hispanic women are still substantial. It is estimated that each year 1.5 million women in the U.S. suffer fractures caused by OP, including 350,000 hip fractures. OP is a severely disabling condition; 70% of those afflicted with the condition do not resume their pre-injury functioning (American Association of Orthopaedic Surgeons, 1999). Up to 20% of women who sustain a hip fracture die within one year (Gass and Dawson-Hughes, 2006; Daly and Carr, 2004).

The incidence of OP fractures increases with age and is more prevalent in women (Maravic, et al., 2005). Women, aged 65 years and older, especially those aged 85 years and older, are susceptible to OP (Gass and Dawson-Hughes, 2006). The age-adjusted rate of OP is 17.3 per 1,000 standard population 65 years and older (U.S. Department of Health & Human Services-Public Health Service, 2002). OP also occurs in men. With the aging of the developed world's population, OP will increase in prevalence, requiring multiple treatment interventions and prevention programs (Franck, et al., 2005).

In some instances, OP vertebral fractures produce deformities of the vertebral column and increase the likelihood of mortality (Miazgowski, 2005). Hasserius, et al. (2005)'s follow-up study of women and men with vertebral fracture showed that women who had a new vertebral fracture at a 12-year follow-up had a higher subsequent mortality rate in the next 10 years, compared to women without a new vertebral fracture. In addition, in a 22-year follow-up, the mortality rate for women with a vertebral fracture was higher than for the female population at risk. The mortality rate was also higher for men with a vertebral fracture, compared to the male population at risk.

A majority of individuals with OP have bone loss (Wilkins and Birge, 2005). Three types of vertebral deformity have been identified: crush, wedge, and biconcave deformities (Ismail, et al., 1999).

Based on a study of 13,562 women and men, Ismail, et al. (1999) found that wedge deformities were the most prevalent deformity and tended to cluster at the mid-thoracic and thoraco-lumbar areas of the spine in both women and men. With age, the prevalence of all three types of vertebral deformity increased, and this was more apparent in women than men. Back pain (BP) was related to all types of vertebral deformity.

Using a random population sample in a prospective study, Miazgowski (2005) found that the incidence of OP vertebral deformity was similar among women (12.6%) and men (10.3%).

However, men in the 50-64 year age group had a significantly higher incidence compared to women but after 4 years, women had a higher prevalence of new vertebral fractures.

In a 12-year follow-up study of 187 elderly women and 70 elderly men with vertebral fracture in the thoracic or lumbar spine, Hasserius, et al. (2005) showed that women had a higher incidence of new vertebral fractures than men.

Fibromyalgia (FM)

Estimates of the prevalence of fibromyalgia (FM) vary. According to the American College of Rheumatology, the disease afflicts 3 to 6 million Americans (http://www.wrongdiagnosis.com/f/fibromyalia/prevalence.htm). According to the National Fibromyalgia Association, an estimated 10 million persons in the U.S. suffer from FM. About 5% of the world's population has this condition (National Fibromyalgia Association, 2006).

FM is more prevalent in women. However, it afflicts men, women, and children in every age group and racial/ethnic background (National Fibromyalgia Association, 2006).

Various reports have shown that the disease often afflicts older individuals (Gowin, 2000; Wolfe, et al., 1995; Holland and Gonzalez, 1998). Based on a random sample of 3,006 individuals in Wichita, Kansas, Wolfe, et al. (1995) found that the prevalence of FM increased with age. In their study, the highest prevalence of FM occurred in the 60-79 year age group.

Based on a sample of three age groups (20-39 years, 40-59 years, and 60-85 years), Cronan, et al. (2002) discovered that symptom duration increased with increasing age. However, the symptoms of the disease were not exacerbated in the older population. The investigation also revealed that psychosocial conditions in the varying age groups had no impact on mediating FM associated pain.

Data from the London Fibromyalgia Epidemiology Study revealed that persons with the disease had the same mean age (47.8 years, range 19 to 86 years) as those of the persons without the disease (White, 1999). However, among individuals with the condition, females were older and reported more symptoms than males.

Rustoen, et al. (2005) evaluated the experience of chronic pain, including that of FM. His study was based on a survey of Norwegian citizens in three age groups (young adults, 18-39 years; middle-aged, 40-59 years; and older adults, 60-81 years). The findings showed that middle-aged persons reported having FM more often than 18-39 year-olds and older adults. The middle-aged individuals were more likely to report that the cause of their pain was unknown.

Low Back Pain (LBP)

Low back pain (LBP) probably afflicts most people in all societies and ethnic groups and at some time (about 20% annually) (Ehrlich, 2003). A review of the literature by Bressler, et al. (1999) showed that the prevalence of LBP in older individuals varies widely in different studies. D'Astolfo and Humphreys (2006) found that the prevalence of BP varies between 36% and 40%. Based on data from the National Health Interview Survey, 27% of adults reported having LBP in 2003 (USDHHS, Health, United States, 2005). LBP was slightly more prevalent among women than men.

According to the National Health Interview Survey, the prevalence of LBP in 2003 increased with age (USDHHS, Health, United States, 2005). The prevalence of LBP peaked among men aged 45 to 64 years (30%) and then decreased in the 65 years and older age group (about 25%). Among women, the prevalence of LBP was similar in both middle-aged and older women (about 32% in both age groups).

Dionne, et al. (2006), in their systematic review of population-based studies, discovered that the prevalence of severe types of BP increased with age. However, the prevalence of benign and mixed back problems did fit the curvilinear association between age and BP symptoms that is found in some studies. They also noted that the evidence concerning the prevalence of BP with age is scarce.

Based on data from the Jerusalem Longitudinal Study, Jacobs, et al. (2006) evaluated 277 persons, aged 70 years at the start of the study and then again at age 77 years. Their results showed that the prevalence of chronic BP increased from 44% at age 70 years to 58% at age 77 years.

Hartvigsen, et al. (2004), in a population-based study of 4,486 Danish twins, aged 70-102 years, found that the overall 1-month prevalence of BP was 15%. They discovered that the prevalence of concurrent back and neck pain was 11% and the prevalence of neck pain alone was 11%. Their results indicated that the prevalence did not vary significantly over time or between age groups.

The prevalence of LBP may depend on whether it is acute, e.g., having disabling LBP for less than 3 months or chronic, having functionally limiting LBP for 3 months or longer. Carey, et al. (1996) studied acute, severe LBP using a population-based telephone interview survey of 4,437 households in North Carolina. Their findings showed that 7.6% of the persons studied had acute severe LBP. Persons who were older than 60 years were less likely to report acute LBP than younger persons (5% compared to 8.5%). Acute LBP was less prevalent in nonwhites compared to whites (5% vs. 8.5%).

The prevalence of LBP in older populations may vary depending on whether the study participants are living in the community or institutionalized. Based on a review of the literature, Fox, et al. (1999) discovered that BP was a predominant painful condition in older adults in nursing homes and other long-term care institutions. Likewise, joints and backs were some of the common sites of pain in nursing home residents in rural New South Wales (McClean and Higginbotham, 2002). In their investigation of musculoskeletal pain in long-term care residents in Ontario, D'Astolfo and Humphreys (2006) showed that 21% of the residents reported BP and 2% reported neck pain.

Despite the studies that have been conducted, definitive knowledge about LBP is lacking and it is believed that its prevalence in older populations is under reported (Dionne, et al., 2006; Bressler, 1999). Co-morbidity in aged populations and problems in research methods increase the variability in the reported prevalence rates.

Cardiovascular Disease

Heart disease and stroke are the most prevalent cardiovascular diseases. More than 70 million residents in the U.S., more than one-fourth of the population, have cardiovascular disease (Centers for Disease Control and Prevention, National Center for Chronic Disease Prevention and Health Promotion, 2006). More than 927,000 Americans die annually from cardiovascular disease or stroke, which is 1 death every 24 seconds. These mostly preventable diseases are more prevalent among individual aged 65 years or older.

Hypertension and high blood cholesterol are two major independent risk factors for cardiovascular disease (Centers for Disease Control and Prevention, National Center for Chronic Disease Prevention and Health Promotion). It is estimated that in 2000 there were more than 972 million individuals who had hypertension worldwide (Chockalingam, et al., 2006). This number is expected to increase to more than 1.56 billion by 2025.

It was reported that between 1999 and 2002, almost 29% of adults in the U.S. had hypertension. Of these individuals, 45% were being treated with medication, but only 29% had their hypertension under control (Centers for Disease Control and Prevention, National Center for Chronic Disease Prevention and Health Promotion). It is estimated that a 12- to 13-point reduction in blood pressure can reduce the risk of myocardial infarctions by 21%, strokes by 37%, and all cardiovascular disease-associated deaths by 25%.

Between 1999 and 2002, approximately 25% of American adults had high cholesterol levels or were being treated with medication (Centers for Disease Control and Prevention, National Center for Chronic Disease Prevention and Health Promotion). Among those with high cholesterol levels, only 63% were aware of it. It is interesting to note that a 10% reduction in cholesterol levels may decrease the incidence of coronary heart disease by as much as 30%.

Kosiborod, et al. (2006), analyzed a national sample of 3,957,520 Medicare beneficiaries, aged 65 years or older, who were hospitalized with heart failure between 1992 and 1999. They discovered no major reductions in mortality and hospital readmissions. More in-depth research is needed to determine the extent to which the recent substantial cardiovascular advancements have had on mortality, heart failure and hospital admission rates.

CHD is a major cause of early, permanent impairment among American workers (Centers for Disease Control and Prevention, National Center for Chronic Disease Prevention and Health Promotion, 2006). Stroke by itself is responsible for disability among approximately 1 millions residents in the U.S.

Cancer

Worldwide, cancer deaths are increasing. It is estimated that by 2020 the number of cancer deaths could reach 10 million (American Cancer Society, 2006, Press Room). A majority of these deaths will occur in developing countries, where the medical care is substandard.

In the U.S., there were an estimated 1.4 million new cases of cancer diagnosed in 2006. (American Cancer Society, Inc., 2006). This estimate does not include non-melanoma skin cancer cases. Cancer is the second leading cause of death in the U.S. About 570,280 Americans or more than 1,500 persons per day died from cancer in 2005 (Centers for Disease Control and Prevention, National Center for Chronic Disease Prevention and Health Promotion, 2006). In 2006, there were an estimated 212,920 new female breast cancer cases, 148,610 new colon and rectum cancer cases, and 174,470 new lung and bronchus cancer cases (American Cancer Society, Inc., 2006).

The probability of developing invasive cancers increases with age (American Cancer Society, Inc., 2006). Between 2000 and 2002, about 39.6% of men and 26.7% of women, aged 70 years and older, had the probability of developing invasive cancers at all cancer sites. In contrast, only about 8.6% of men and 9.1% of women, aged 40 to 59 years, had the chance of developing invasive cancers at all cancer sites. About 7.1% of women, aged 70 years and older, had a probability of developing invasive breast cancer, whereas about 4.1% of women, aged 40 to 59 years, had a probability of developing invasive breast cancer. About 4.9% of men and 4.6% of women, aged 70 years and older have a probability of developing invasive colorectal cancer, compared to less than 1% of men and less than 1% of women, aged 40 to 59 years. More than 6% of men and about 4% of women, aged 70 years and older have a chance of developing invasive cancer of the lung and bronchus, compared to 1% of men and less than 1% of women, aged 40 to 59 years.

In 2002, the three most prevalent and deadly cancers among men were: prostate cancer, lung cancer, and colorectal cancer (Centers for Disease Control and Prevention, Cancer-U.S. Cancer Statistics, 2002).

The leading causes of death among men were: 1. lung cancer; 2. prostate cancer among white, African-American, and Hispanic men, whereas prostate cancer was third among American Indian/Alaska natives; 3. Colorectal cancer was the third leading cause of cancer death among white, African-American, Asian/Pacific Islander, and Hispanic men but was second among American Indian/Alaska natives.

The three most prevalent cancers among women were: breast cancer, lung cancer, and colorectal cancer. Breast cancer was the most prevalent type of cancer among women of all racial and Hispanic-origin groups (Centers for Disease Control and Prevention, Cancer-U.S. Cancer Statistics, 2002).

Lung cancer, breast cancer, and colorectal cancer were the three leading causes of cancer death among women in 2002 (Centers for Disease Control and Prevention, Cancer-U.S. Cancer Statistics, 2002).

Lifestyle and Behavioral Factors

Lifestyle and behavioral factors are responsible for a variety of chronic diseases and associated morbidity and mortality trends. In the U.S., about 45.8 million adults smoke cigarettes. Each year, tobacco use will result in about 440,000 deaths (Centers for Disease Control and Prevention, National Center for Chronic Disease Prevention and Health Promotion, 2006).

Older adults who try to quit smoking often have multiple relapses (Andrews, et al., 2004). Aged adult smokers tend to have less education, low socioeconomic status, and are more likely to be women. Older adult smokers also tend to have low levels of self-efficacy regarding smoking cessation.

Aged adult smokers are more likely than younger smokers to suffer from smoking-associated diseases (Andrews, et al., 2004). However, they experience similar benefits from smoking cessation as younger smokers. Andrews, et al. (2004) notes that aged adults often want to stop smoking and do so at similar rates as younger smokers. The authors recommend that treating smoking dependence in aged adults should have the same emphasis as treating other chronic diseases in this population. They note that clinicians can be effective in treating smoking dependence regardless of the smoker's age or smoking history. Treatment should consist of pharmacological and behavioral therapies plus health care intervention to help older patients reduce their tobacco use. More research is needed, however, to assess the effectiveness of smoking cessation interventions on older adults (Doolan and Froelicher, 2006).

Please note that while the statistics cited in the following two paragraphs refer to adults, in general, these problems also pertain to the older adults. Sedentary lifestyles, poor nutritional habits, and inadequate psychosocial adaptation to life stresses lead to increased rates of obesity and associated diseases. Obesity rates among adults doubled between 1980 and 2000. About 30% of the adult population or 60 million adults are currently obese. It is estimated that obesity is responsible for about 112,000 deaths annually in the U.S. (Centers for Disease Control and Prevention, National Center for Chronic Disease Prevention and Health Promotion, 2006).

Lock, et al. (2005) estimated that that up to 2.635 million deaths annually are due to low consumption of fruit and vegetables. They found that consumption of fruit and vegetables to up to 600 g per day could lower total worldwide disease burden by 1.8% and lower the burden of ischemic heart disease and ischemic stroke by 31% and 19%, respectively. This nutritional goal could reduce the burden of stomach, esophageal, lung, and colorectal cancer by 19%, 20%, 12%, and 2%, respectively.

Manini, et al. (2006) evaluated energy expenditure in 302 high functioning adults, aged, 70 to 82 years. They found that those who were the most physically active had significantly lower chances of dying than those with the lowest physical activity level.

Maraldi, et al., using information from a sample of adults aged 70 to 79 from the Health, Aging and Body Composition (HABC) study, found that persons drinking 1 to 7 alcohol drinks per week had lower age-, sex-, and race-adjusted incidences of death, compared with those who never or only occasionally drank alcohol (20.1 vs. 27.4 per 1000 person-years, respectively).

However, there is still uncertainty about the survival benefit of alcohol use and the processes underlying the protective impact of light to moderate alcohol consumption. Recent data suggests that light to moderate alcohol use has an anti-inflammatory effect. For instance, using data from the HABC investigation, Volpato, et al. (2004) revealed that light alcohol use is linked to lower levels of interleukin-6 and C-reactive protein. However, they found no link between alcohol consumption and tumor necrosis factor-alpha and plasminogen activator inhibtor-1.

Stress reduction strategies have been shown to have significant psychosocial benefit and may be helpful in reducing morbidity and mortality in older adults (Taylor-Piliae, et al., 2006; Schneider, et al., 2005). For example, participation in mind-body exercise, such as Tai Chi, has been associated with improvements in emotional well-being, stress-reduction, and mental health. Schneider, et al.

(2005) evaluated the long-term effects of stress reduction on mortality in adults, aged 55 years or older, with systemic hypertension. Based on pooled data from two published randomized controlled trials that included a Transcendental Meditation (TM) program, other behavioral interventions, and usual care, the authors found that participants in the TM group had a 23% reduction in the rate of all-cause mortality, a 30% reduction in cardiovascular mortality, and a 49% reduction in cancer-related mortality, compared with controls. The researchers conclude that TM, as a stress-reducing approach in the prevention and control of high blood pressure, may help to reduce all-cause mortality as well as cardiovascular disease mortality in this population.

Air Pollution and Other Environmental Hazards

As people age, they are less able to compensate for the impact of air pollution and other environmental hazards (AirNow, 2006, http://airnow.gov/index.cfm). Studies have shown that air pollution can worsen cardiovascular disease and stroke, chronic pulmonary disease, and diabetes. As a consequence, older adults who are exposed to significant air pollution are likely to use more medications, visit their health care providers more often, have more emergency room visits and hospital admissions, and have a higher death rate than those not exposed to high levels of air pollution.

Older people are especially vulnerable to ozone and particulate matter (PM), especially fine particle pollution known as PM 2.5 (AirNow, 2006, http://airnow.gov/index.cfm). Research has shown that fine particle pollution increases the risk of premature death, cardiac arrhythmias and heart attacks, asthma attacks, and chronic bronchitis. Even at low levels, ozone has been found to worsen pulmonary diseases.

2
Elders and Health Care Utilization and Costs

Health Care Utilization

Older adults use a wide range of health care services at a higher rate than other age groups. For example, seniors spend more time in hospitals than younger persons. An analysis of short-stay hospitals showed that persons, 75 years of age and older, had an average length of stay (ALOS) of 6.8 days, individuals in the 65 to 74 year age group had an ALOS of 5.9 days, those 45 to 64 years of age had an ALOS of 4.5 days, and persons 18-44 years of age had an ALOS of 3.5 days (USDHHS, Health, United States, 2002; Shi and Singh, 2004).

Seniors have more ambulatory office visits than younger persons. A study of the rate of national ambulatory office visits revealed that individuals in the 65-74 year age group had 5.8 visits per year, those 75 years of age and older had 6.5 visits per year, compared to persons in the 25-44 year age group who had 2.4 visits per year (USDHHS, 2002; Shi and Singh, 2004).

In addition, most long-term care services (a range of health care, mental health, social support, and residential services, including home health care, adult day care, hospice care, assisted living facilities, skilled nursing facilities, subacute care facilities, and continuing care retirement communities) are used by persons age 65 years and older (Shi and Singh, 2004).

Neither age nor diagnosis of a disease can completely determine if a person will need long-term care services. In fact, the prevalence of chronic disability among seniors has declined in recent decades (Manton and Gu, 2001). Nevertheless, with the aging boom, the elderly population's growing need for long-term care services is expected to place severe financial pressures on a shrinking group of working taxpayers. To help control costs and maintain quality of care, case management services are used to coordinate the wide variety of potential long-term care services available for seniors and help reduce unnecessary and duplicated services (Shi and Singh, 2004).

With the aging of the baby boomers, Medicare costs are expected to increase significantly in the future. To address the spiraling costs of Medicare, the Balanced Budget Act of 1997 mandated the development of Medicare + Choice program (also known as Part C), which allows Medicare beneficiaries to enroll in either a managed care (MC) plan, such as a health maintenance organizations (HMO) or Preferred Provider Organizations (PPO) or a private fee-for-service plan (FFS) (Shi and Singh, 2004). The Medicare + Choice program primarily enrolls beneficiaries with lower income.

Initially, there was growth in the enrollment of Medicare beneficiaries in managed plans (Shi and Singh, 2004). However, since 1999, many MC care plans have terminated their participation in the program. Inadequate Medicare payments have been one of the primary reasons for their withdrawal from Medicare Part C. At the present time, about 11% of all Medicare beneficiaries participate in this program.

Because of limited health care resources and increased costs, one major concern is that health care will be rationed based on age. Since the development of MC, some experts fear that MC organizations, along with physicians at the bedside, may withhold or delay treatment for the elderly and other vulnerable patients (Soumerai, et al., 1999; Kapp, 2002; Churchill, 2005; Ubel, 2001; O'Malley, 1991). A related moral-ethical and social issue deals with the desirability of using expensive life-extending procedures, such as dialysis and transplants, for older adults (Kaufman, et al., 2006; Rodriguez and Young, 2006). Experts are evaluating the extent to which life-sustaining procedures extend life, enhance quality of life, maintain or improve biological functioning, and assist patients on a short-term basis (Rodriguez and Young, 2006). Some rationing plans have been formulated which consider chronological age. However, Kapp (2002) points out that it is unlikely that these schemes will be adopted because of ethical and political factors.

To address concerns over utilization of health resources and quality of care for seniors, investigators have compared health care utilization and quality of care outcomes for Medicare recipients in MC plans and FFS plans. These investigations have yielded mixed results (Retchin, et al., 1997). Retchin, et al. (1997) analyzed health care utilization and survival patterns for stroke patients in MC programs compared to fee-for-service programs. Based on samples of 402 HMO patients from 71 hospitals and 408 FFS patients, the authors discovered HMO patients had a higher probability of being sent to a nursing home than FFS patients following a stroke. HMO patients were also less likely to be sent to a rehabilitation facility than FFS patients. However, at follow-up, there were no significant differences in the relative risk of dying between HMO and FFS patients.

Ware, et al. (1996) used data from the Medical Outcomes Study to compare physical and mental health outcomes of chronically ill seniors and other patients treated in HMO and FFS settings. They found that Medicare patients in HMOs were more likely to have significant declines in physical health than those in FFS settings. Mental health outcomes were better for Medicare patients in HMOs compared to those FFS systems at one site, but these findings were not evident at two other sites.

Soumerai, et al. (1999) compared the timeliness and quality of care for elderly patients with acute myocardial infarction (AMI) in HMOs and FFS settings using a sample of 2,304 Medicare patients who were admitted to 20 urban community hospitals in Minnesota. The authors found that timeliness and quality of care were the same for HMO patients with AMI compared to FFS patients and that two measures of quality of care, use of emergency transportation and aspirin treatment, were slightly better for HMO patients than for FFS patients.

Drug therapy is one of the most effective interventions for improving health outcomes. However, some medications are less appropriate for older patients (Monane, 1998). The toxic effects of prescription and over-the-counter (OTC) medications have major adverse health effects and can lead to excess health care utilization and increased costs (Roumie and Griffin, 2004; Goulding, 2004; Fick, et al., 2003). For example, seniors who use OTC analgesics on a long-term basis, may use excessively high doses, which can result in the development of gastrointestinal hemorrhage, cardiac, kidney and liver toxicity (Roumie and Griffin, 2004). In addition, the concurrent use of pain medications, alcohol, hypertension drugs, and regular caffeine use may result in adverse risks (Amoako, et al., 2003).

To assist emergency physicians in prescribing safe and effective medications for seniors, Terrell, et al. (2006) reviewed the risks related in the use of non-steroidal anti-inflammatory drugs, benzodiazepines, and anticholinergic medications. They found that these drugs may produce adverse outcomes and should be prescribed with caution.

Fick, et al. (2003) used the results of a U.S. consensus panel of experts to update the widely used and cited Beers criteria for potentially inappropriate drug use in adults 65 years and older. The authors identified 48 separate drugs or classes of drugs to avoid in the treatment of 20 diseases or conditions. Sixty-six of these specific drugs had highly severe adverse outcomes. The authors suggest that using the Beers criteria and related procedures would help reduce medication-associated costs, overall health care costs, and medication-related problems.

Goulding (2004) used data from the large scale National Ambulatory Medical Care Survey to determine the extent of inappropriate medication prescribing to elderly for pain relievers and central nervous system drugs, e.g., anti-anxiety drugs, sedatives, and antidepressants. The probability of prescribing inappropriate drugs at these visits increased with multiple drugs and doubled for women.

A study of inappropriate medication use by elderly persons in 10 HMOs in 2000-2001 revealed that 28.8% of the patients were prescribed at least one of 33 potentially inappropriate drugs (Simon, et al., 2005). Across the 10 HMOs, this rate ranged from 23.0% to 36.5%. The results indicated that about 5% of the seniors were prescribed at least one of the 11 drugs categorized by an expert panel as "always avoid," 13% were prescribed at least one of the 8 drugs that would rarely be regarded as appropriate, and 17% were prescribed at least one of 14 drugs that are appropriate but are frequently misused. Women in this study were more likely than men to be prescribed inappropriate drugs.

Older adults are also at high risk of mismanaging their medications (Curry, et al., 2005). The most prevalent types of medication errors made by seniors include combining OTC and prescription drugs, discontinuing essential prescriptions, using incorrect doses, using inappropriate methods of drug administration, and eating the wrong food with their medications.

There are a number of human and environmental factors that increase seniors' risk of self-management errors (Curry, et al., 2005). First, they take more prescription and OTC medications than any other age group (Curry, et al., 2005; Amoako, et al., 2003).

Second, older adults, who are often on fixed incomes tend to self-medicate with OTC because they are cheaper than the more expensive prescription medications (Amoako, et al., 2003). As more drugs become available as OTC medications, as the population ages, and as the prevalence of chronic diseases increases, there will be an increased risk of adverse drug effects in this population.

Third, older adults may stop using high priced prescription medications because they cannot afford them. This is especially true for those with chronic diseases such as diabetes, hypertension, cardiovascular disease, and cancer, who must take a number of medications daily.

Fourth, they may be confused by complicated drug regimes involving drugs with different doses, times of administration, and methods of administration (Curry, et al., 2005).

Fifth, patients frequently have insufficient knowledge about their medications (Curry, et al., 2005). Studies of the general population have found that more than 60% of individuals are unable to identify the active ingredient in their pain medication, and approximately 40% of Americans believe that OTC medications are harmless (Roumie and Griffin, 2004).

Sixth, older adults are at risk for cognitive, sensory, and motor deficits which impair their ability to take prescription and OTC medications properly (Curry, et al., 2005).

Seventh, alcohol-drug interactions and use of complementary and alternative remedies can lead to adverse effects (Curry, et al., 2005). Sleath, et al. (2001) conducted a study of 27 resident physicians and 205 of their Hispanic and non-Hispanic white patients age 50 years and older, and found that almost 18% of the patients reported using one or more alternative treatments during the previous month. The most commonly used treatment was herbal medicine.

Eighth, communication problems between the health care practitioner and patient can contribute to medication errors (Curry, et al., 2005). In some cases the physicians may be unaware that some of their patients are cognitively impaired. In other cases, patients may not inform their physicians that they are using complementary and alternative medicines (CAM). Sleath, et al. (2001) discovered that 83% of patients who had used an alternative treatment in the previous month did not inform their physicians about it. In only 3.4% of office visits did physicians ask one or more questions about their patients' use of CAM. Only 2% of patients asked their clinicians one or more questions about CAM.

Ninth, polypharmacy or the concurrent prescription of multiple medications for seniors increases the risk of medication errors (Curry, et al., 2005). Age-related and disease-related changes in drug absorption, distribution, elimination, and clearance in older adults may increase the risk of adverse consequences from polypharmacy, medication errors, and mismanagement (von Moltke, et al., 2000; Herrlinger and Klotz, 2001).

Tenth, improper storage of medications will result in ineffective medications.

Finally, the lack of clearly marked expiration dates on drugs increases the risk that patients will continue to take medications that are no longer efficacious (Curry, et al., 2005).

A number of strategies can help reduce medication errors and mismanagement in older adults. Terrell, et al. (2006) suggest that opioids, although not without risks, are safe with slow titration, the use of precautions, and constipation treatment. They recommend estimating creatinine clearance when prescribing drugs that necessitate dosage adjustment in patients with potential or actual renal insufficiency. They also urge that more research be undertaken to determine the correct dosing and safety of drugs for older patients. Moreover, the authors recommend more research to determine if prescribing with electronic decision support will help physicians in their prescribing decisions.

Improved patient and health provider education can reduce the risk of medication problems (Curry, et al., 2005; Bergman-Evans, 2006; Joanna Briggs Institute, 2006; Roumie and Griffin, 2004; Amoako, et al., 2003; Goulding, 2004). Curry, et al. (2005) recommends that nurses take advantage of formal and informal teaching opportunities to ensure that patients are thoroughly assessed in terms of their abilities to administer their medications safely. Bergman-Evans (2006) advocates the use of the AIDES method: Assessment that is comprehensive, Individualization of the therapy, Documentation that is appropriate, Education that is customized to the patient's age, and Supervision which is continued after initiation of the treatment.

Online drug utilization review linked to a telephone pharmacy alert may help physicians reduce medication errors (Simon, et al., 2006; Monane, et al., 1998). Simon, et al. (2006) found that age-specific alerts maintained the effectiveness of drug-specific alerts in reducing the number of potentially inappropriate prescriptions for seniors. In addition, written feedback to physicians about medication discrepancies may help physicians correct medication discrepancies, such as patients not taking their charted medications, patients taking medications that were not charted, and errors in drug dosage and schedule (Forjuoh, et al., 2005).

Enhanced labeling of medications can help patients better understand the active ingredients, adverse effects, and contraindications of their medications (Roumie and Griffin, 2004).

Another important component of health care utilization is surgery, and with improvements in surgery, longer life expectancy, and improved surgical outcomes, seniors are increasingly being referred for certain types of surgical operations (USDHH, Health, United States, 2005; Kolh, et al., 2001). For example, for adults age 75 years and older, the rate of hospitalization for coronary stent insertion procedures increased three-fold from 23 per 10,000 population in 1996-97 to 73 in 2002-03 (USDHH, Health, United States, 2005). The rate of hospitalization for this procedure more than doubled for adults age 65-74 from about 35 per 10,000 population in 1996-97 to about 80 in 2002-2005.

As surgery has been extended into older populations, health-related quality of life (HRQL) has been used as an important indicator of surgical success (Hornick, 2006). HRQL measures can be used to determine the appropriateness of surgery for seniors who face substantial surgery-related morbidity and mortality. New techniques, such as laparoscopic or minimally invasive surgery, have great potential for reducing perioperative problems and improving HRQL in younger age groups. However, these techniques have not been used extensively in older age groups, who may derive even greater potential benefits from these procedures than younger age groups.

Health Care Costs

A significant amount of health care expenditures are for Medicare beneficiaries (persons 65 years of age and over and disabled persons). In 2003, 30% of hospital expenditures were paid by Medicare (USDHH, Health, United States, 2005). However, Medicare paid only 12% of nursing home care in 2003. Despite the availability of Medicare, seniors may still have substantial out-of-pocket health care expenditures. This is particularly true for those with poor health and higher total expenditures and individuals with significant prescription medication expenses since drug expenses are less likely to be covered by health insurance than hospital and physician expenses. More than 40% of non-institutionalized adults, aged 65 years and older with medical expenses spent at least $1,000 out-of-pocket in 2002.

The costs of chronic diseases consist of both direct medical costs and indirect costs such as lost workdays and reduced productivity. However, it is difficult to calculate total health care costs for non-employed elderly since in the general population the calculations of indirect costs involve determining changes in work status (Katz, 2006).

It is difficult to evaluate the true costs of care to the non-employed older population because few studies deal with them. I have, therefore, considered the problems as studied in the broader population in order to obtain some estimates of the probable costs for the elderly.

Estimates of the costs of chronic diseases underestimate the true burden of these diseases since they may omit the costs associated with pain and suffering, the care given by family and other caregivers, and the services of other health providers that are necessitated by the patient's chronic condition (Hogan, et al., 2003). Nevertheless, the direct and indirect costs of chronic diseases are enormous.

Diabetes Mellitus (DM)

Diabetes mellitus (DM) costs are increasing worldwide (Logminiene, et al., 2004). Between 1969 and 1997, the direct medical costs of DM increased from 1.7 billion U.S. dollars to 44.4 billion U.S. dollars. Indirect DM costs during this period increased from 1.6 billion U.S. dollars to 54.1 billion U.S. dollars.

In 2002, the total economic costs of DM in the U.S. were estimated to be $132 billion (Hogan, et al., 2003; Centers for Disease Control and Prevention, National Center for Chronic Disease Prevention and Health Promotion). The total direct medical costs were $91.8 billion dollars. DM care accounted for about 23.1 billion dollars, chronic complications accounted for 24.6 billion dollars, and increased prevalence of general medical conditions accounted for 44.1 billion dollars (Hogan, et al., 2003). Major DM expenditures consist of hospitalizations (43.9%), nursing home care (15.1%), and office visits (10.9%). Persons over age 65 years incurred 51.8% of direct medical costs. The total indirect costs of DM, such as the number of days away from work, number of days of restricted activity, and impairment associated with the condition were about $39.8 billion dollars.

Certain older diabetics face risks of financial burdens. The greatest financial burden is borne by those with private non-employment-associated insurance; then come those who have Medicare only; they are followed by those with employment-associated coverage; and then those with the least financial burden – the Medicaid beneficiaries. The second greatest financial burdens are faced by older diabetics who have Medicare only, followed by those with employment-associated coverage. Among aged persons, 62% to 69% of out-of-pocket expenditures are for prescription medications and diabetic supplies (Bernard, et al., 2006).

Arthritis

Arthritis is a leading cause of impairment and results in substantial Social Security disability payments because of chronic absence from work and employment loss (NIH News Release, 1998; National Arthritis Action Plan, 1999). More than 7 million persons in the U.S. are limited in their daily activities because of this disease. Those with more moderate arthritic conditions are not reflected in this number, but still face an economic burden because of their condition. The annual total costs for treating arthritis and disease-related complications and for the disabilities that are produced by these disorders are almost $65 billion dollars. Almost $15 billion dollars of the costs come from 39 million physician visits and more than half a million hospitalizations (About Arthritis).

Rheumatoid Arthritis (RA)

Researchers have evaluated the costs related to specific forms of arthritis. For example, Birnbaum, et al. (2000) analyzed the annual per capita costs of rheumatoid arthritis (RA) for beneficiaries of a large employer. The authors showed that the annual per capita employer costs for RA employees who were impaired were almost three times those of controls ($17,822 dollars vs. $6,131 dollars).

Osteoporosis (OP)

The costs of osteoporosis (OP) to society are substantial. The acute and long-term medical care costs of treating OP fractures in the U.S. are estimated to be between $10 billion dollars to $18 billion dollars (Keen, 2003; American Association of Orthopaedic Surgeons, 1999). Hip fractures generate the largest OP-associated health care costs. The repair and rehabilitation of a hip fracture costs about $16,000 dollars (Burge, et al., 1997). A study of OP fractures in France also revealed that median in-patient costs were higher for hip fractures (8,048 to 8,727 Euros) than for fractures of the humerus (3,786 Euros) and radius (2,363 to 2,574 Euros) (Maravic, et al., 2005). Because of the dramatic aging of the population and the increase in the incidence of OP fractures in younger age groups, the disease is considered a major public health problem (American Association of Orthopaedic Surgeons, 1999).

Fibromyalgia (FM)

Fibromyalgia (FM) poses a huge economic and social burden to both the individual and society. It is estimated that the annual FM costs in the U.S. are between $12 billion to $14 billion. About 1 to 2% of the nation's lost productivity is due to the condition (National Fibromyalgia Association, 2006).

Robinson, et al. (2003) investigated the economic cost of FM using administrative claims data of a Fortune 100 manufacturer. They compared 4,699 patients with at least one FM claim between 1996 and 1996 and a 10% random sample of the total beneficiary population. The results of their study showed that the prevalence of disability among employees with FM was two times as high as among all employees. The total annual costs for FM claimants were more than twice as high as the costs for the typical beneficiary ($5,945 vs. $2,486). For every dollar the employer spent on FM claims, they spent another $57 to $143 on additional direct and indirect costs.

Low Back Pain (LBP)

The total costs of low back pain (LBP) in the U.S. are more than $100 billion dollars annually (Katz, 2006). Of this amount, two thirds are indirect, resulting from lost employment and decreased productivity. Annually, less than 5% of the patients with LBP make up 75% of the total costs. The substantial costs associated with LBP are reflected in the large number of office visits made for the treatment of BP. In 2003, adults, aged 18 years and older, made 3.6 million visits to physician offices and hospital outpatient facilities for treatment of BP (USDHHS, Health, United States, 2005). Office visits and hospital outpatient departments for BP account for only a portion of total health care costs for this condition since they only include persons who have used the health care system. Additional medical costs are incurred by individuals who self-treat BP with OTC medications and CAM.

Weiner, et al. (2006), using outpatient national and Pennsylvania Part A Medicare beneficiary data related to non-invasive or minimally invasive evaluation and treatment of non-specific LBP, discovered that between 1991 and 2002, there was a 42.5% increase in total Medicare patients and a 131.7% increase in patients with LBP. During this same period there was a 310% increase in total charges and a 387.2% in charges related to LBP. An analysis of Pennsylvania Part A Medicare beneficiary data between 2000 and 2002 revealed that there was a 5.5% increase in patients with LBP and 33.2% increase in LBP charges. The investigators also discovered that out of 111 older adults with chronic LBP who were interviewed, 61% had MRIs (29% with neurogenic claudication and 24% with failed back surgery), although none of them had "red flags" or indications that necessitated imaging. The authors conclude that in Medicare beneficiaries, documentation of LBP and related diagnostic studies are increasing. In addition, they suggest that MRIs may frequently be undertaken unnecessarily. A significant proportion of the LBP-related costs are for injection and imaging procedures

A study conducted in the Netherlands found that the costs were higher for chronic low back pain (CLBP) (8,533 Euros) and FM (7, 813 Euros) than for ankylosing spondylitis (3,205 Euros) (Boonen, et al., 2005). The study also revealed that the level of well-being was lower in patients with FM and CLBP than in patients with ankylosing spondylitis.

Cardiovascular Disease

In 2006, the total direct and indirect economic cost of heart disease and stroke in the U.S. is estimated to be $403 billion dollars, including health expenditures and lost productivity from disability and death (Centers for Disease Control and Prevention, National Center for Chronic Disease Prevention and Health Promotion). The estimated direct and indirect cost of hypertension in 2006 is $64 billion dollars. It is estimated that more than 6 million hospitalizations annually are due to cardiovascular disease.

The concurrent prescription of multiple medications for older heart disease patients increases the costs of health care. Masoudi, et al. (2005) evaluated the chronic medications prescribed at hospital discharge to patients, aged 65 years or older, hospitalized for heart failure (HF). The authors discovered that between 1998 and 1999, the mean number of drugs prescribed was 6.8. This represented 10.1 doses daily at a cost of $3,142 dollars annually. In 2000 to 2001, the mean number of drugs increased to 7.5, with 11.1 doses daily at a cost of $3,823 dollars. A number of factors were predictive of the increased complexity and costs of health care for HF patients: having DM, previous revascularization, and chronic pulmonary disease.

The Screening for Heart Attack Prevention and Education (SHAPE) Task Force suggests that mass cardiovascular screening of American men over 45 years of age and most women over 55 could prevent 90,000 deaths from heart attack each year (Naghavi, et al., 2006; Edelson, 2006). The SHAPE Task Force recommends that physicians evaluate the arteries of apparently healthy individuals to determine their levels of arterial plaque and the thickness of the wall of the carotid artery, the primary blood vessel leading up the neck to the brain. Plaques consist of fatty deposits that can build up in the arteries, causing heart attack or stroke. The task force estimates that these mass examinations would reduce the number of Americans who have heart attacks, currently estimated at 13.2 million, by 25%. The task force suggests that universal screening would save more than $21.5 billion dollars in health care costs each year by identifying individuals at risk much sooner than they are identified now.

Cancer

The total cancer cost in 2004 was estimated to be $189 billion dollars (Centers for Disease Control and Prevention, National Center for Chronic Disease Prevention and Health Promotion). Of this amount, direct medical costs amounted to $69 billion dollars and indirect costs such as lost work-days and productivity amounted to $120 billion dollars.

The costs of cancer to employers in the U.S. can be significant. A case-control study of cancer costs to a large U.S. employer revealed that $224 dollars per active employee or 6.5% of the company's total health care expenditures was spent on the care of cancer patients in 1997 (Barnett et al., 2000). The annual health care and disability costs for cancer patients were about 5 times higher than for those who did not have cancer.

The costs associated with specific cancers have been analyzed. One study using data from 2000 estimated that the costs of treating breast cancer in the U. S. are more than $7 billion dollars per year (Centers for Disease Control and Prevention, The National Breast and Cervical Cancer Early Detection Program, 2006). Redaelli, et al. (2003) estimated that the costs of colorectal cancer in the U.S. were between $5.5 and $6.5 million dollars.

Lifestyle and Behavioral Factors

Lifestyle and unhealthy behaviors create a huge economic and social burden for society. It is estimated that smoking-associated diseases cost more than $155 billion dollars each year (Centers for Disease Control and Prevention, National Center for Chronic Disease Prevention and Health Promotion, 2006). Direct annual costs attributable to tobacco use are more than $75 billion dollars and indirect costs are $80 billion dollars.

The economic and social burden of obesity is also substantial. In 1995, direct health costs associated with obesity were estimated to be $52 billion and this increased to $75 billion in 2003 (Centers for Disease Control and Prevention, National Center for Chronic Disease Prevention and Health Promotion, 2006). Over the past two decades, hospital costs related to overweight and obesity more than tripled.

3
Chronic Disease and Quality of Life in Older Adults

Quality of life has been defined as "the subjective judgment of the net valence of one's life as marked by time intervals from very brief to very long (Magai and McFadden, 1996, pg. 344)." Contributors to the experience of quality of life include temperament, cognitive-affective schemata from past experiences and the intensity of affect. However, quality of life for older people has typically been reduced to quality of life as related to health-related quality of life. Gabriel and Bowling (2004) and Wiggins, et al. (2004) have, both posited that functional status, as well as other subjective dimensions of aging need to be considered. Exactly what constitutes quality of life on a personal level varies from one individual to the next. Some people focus on material possessions, while some focus on achievement. Others may focus on a sense of happiness or well-being.

Although many older adults have good health, most do experience increased physical problems that affect them and their activity level. Furthermore, changes become subtler as people age and they may not be aware of differences. Certainly diseases do occur more frequently with advancing age, including dementia, Alzheimer's disease (AD), arthritis, hypertension, stroke, heart disease, depression, osteoporosis (OP), as well as kidney and bladder problems, lung disease, cancer, and prostate disease in men.

As an individual ages, the person experiences a number of changes, not only physical changes, but sensory changes, cognitive changes and emotional/personality changes as well. Genes and environment, both, determine one's experience of aging. However, Lebow (1998) argued that lifestyle choices most powerfully determine how people age. Diet, exercise, mental stimulation, a sense of self efficacy and connection to others emerged as key factors in maintaining high function and contentment in life.

In a recent study (Strawbridge, et al., 2002), the percentage of those 65-99 years old rating themselves as aging successfully was 50.3%. The absence of chronic conditions and maintaining functioning were positively associated with successful aging. However, many participants in the study with chronic conditions and with functional difficulties still rated themselves as aging successfully.

In another study, Lawton (1999) evaluated 600 healthy and chronically ill elderly individuals aged 70 years and older. They determined that valuation of life was an internal representation of many positive and negative features of the person and his/her everyday life and that this valuation of life impacted quality of life and an individual's will to live or not.

According to the Economic and Social Research Council in the United Kingdom (2003), the quality of life is less influenced by the past and more influenced by the present. In this longitudinal study, a number of factors were related to quality of life. Health and socio-economic factors were found to have a role, in that the quality of life for the affluent-healthy is higher than for the deprived-unhealthy. Furthermore, the study also revealed that the quality of life was better for a healthy, poor person than for a person in poor health. The study also indicated that the quality and density of one's social network was more important than the number of people in one's social sphere and that the neighborhood in which one lives has little impact except in a negative sense (e.g., when there is fear). Finally, control over when to work or retire has a significant impact on quality of life, with the issue of choice paramount.

Rowe and Kahn (1998) studied successful aging, specifically focusing on the impact of specific lifestyle choices on the experience of aging. They discovered that there were a number of factors that contributed to a positive quality of life, including regimens of healthy diet, exercise and health related behaviors (losing weight and stopping smoking).

Crowther, et al. (2002) proposed that there was a missing component to Rowe and Kahn's three-factor model. Their evidence suggested that spirituality was also related to one's experience of aging and concomitantly, the individual's quality of life.

Daviglus, et al. (2003) found that a higher body mass index was associated with a poorer quality of life in older age, as well as higher morbidity and shorter life expectancy. The researchers also discovered that a favorable cardiovascular profile was associated with better quality of life. Crogan and Pasvogel (2003) also found a relationship between body mass index with functional status (eating, personal hygiene and toilet use) and psychosocial well being.

Obesity is a well-known risk factor for a variety of chronic illnesses in older adults, including cardiovascular disease, diabetes mellitus (DM), arthritis, blindness, and amputation (Aldwin and Gilmer, 2004). For example, glucose intolerance usually precedes the onset of DM, resulting in higher blood sugar levels and ultimately damage to the pancreas. In turn, DM contributes to aging of both the sensory and cardiovascular systems and may also affect ambulation. However, diet, weight loss and exercise can reverse glucose intolerance and ameliorate early DM. Knowler, et al. (2002) found that some interventions, including counseling and exercise, decreased or delayed the onset of DM by over 50%, compared to those who utilized drug therapy alone.

Vailas, et al. (1998) reported that quality of life and quality of health were positively related. In addition, they noted that nutritional risk, decreased enjoyment of food, depression and impaired functional status were all negatively associated with quality of life. In another study, Keller, et al. (2004) commented that nutrition parameters have been linked to quality of life, but few studies have determined if nutritional risk predicts changes in quality of life over time in older adults. Their study determined that nutritional risk was in fact an independent predictor of change in health-related quality of life and that there was a relationship between nutrition and the more holistic view of quality of life. Seniors with high nutritional risk had fewer good physical health days and whole-life satisfaction compared with those with low risk. Shibata (2001) studied the nutritional factors in Japanese elderly and found that low serum cholesterol accelerated depression and was associated with lower levels of functional capacity. However, in another study, Strandberg, et al. (2004) found that low serum cholesterol predicted better physical functioning and quality of life in old age, without negatively affecting cognition.

Menec (2003) examined the longitudinal relationship of activity to aging and found that greater overall activity level was related to greater happiness, better function and reduced mortality. Different activities were related to different outcome measures, but social and productive activities were positively related to happiness, function and mortality. By contrast, more solitary activities like hobbies were related only to happiness. Many older people continue to do substantial productive work, whether paid or unpaid. The McArthur Foundation Study of Aging in America (1998) reported that more than 40 percent of the elderly report at least 1,500 hours of productive activity per year. Only 2 percent report not engaging in any type of productive activity. Furthermore, even individuals age 75 and over report providing informal help to friends and relatives, although this informal work reaches its zenith between the ages of 55 and 64.

Exercise can slow down the rate of aging by regulating weight, improving muscle strength and positively effecting cholesterol. Exercise in older adults can improve muscle strength, flexibility, walking and balance (Keysor and Jette, 2001). Exercise tends to improve cardiovascular functioning. Although cardiac output decreases with age, older adults who are physically fit can increase their cardiac output 50% more than those who are not physically fit (Guyton and Hall, 1996). Furthermore, exercise also protects pulmonary functioning. In one study, Puggaard, et al. (2000) found that aerobic exercise could increase vital capacity and VO2 max, even in 85-year-old women.

Psychosocial factors also have a significant role in the older adult's quality of life. There is much evidence that personality affects health, especially cardiovascular health (Aldwin, et al., 2004; Krantz and McCerney, 2001; Smith and Spiro, 2002). There have been a number of studies on hostility and Type A behavior in particular. In 1978, the review panel on coronary-prone behavior and coronary heart disease presented evidence indicating that hostility was comparable to smoking as a risk factor for cardiovascular disease. The effect was found to be stronger for men than for women (Williams, 2000).

Anxiety and depression are also related to the quality of life in older adults. Neuroticism appears to predict mortality independent of hostility (Surtees, et al., 2003). Furthermore, Wilson, et al. (2004) demonstrated that this is particularly true in later life. Anxiety has been found to be associated with higher risks of cardiac disease (Tennant and McLean, 2001) and sudden cardiac death (Kawachi, et al., 1994). With depression, older individuals who recover from depression have a lower risk of mortality (Blazer, 2001). Yet, depression has been associated with higher levels of cardiovascular mortality (Tennat and McLean, 2001).

Surprisingly, research on the effects of optimism on health in older adults has been inconsistent. Some studies have indicated that optimism is related to better self-reported health (Peterson, 1988). In another study, Kubzansky, et al. (2001) showed that optimism was related to a reduction in cardiovascular disease. Giltay, et al. (2004) posited that optimism was consistent with lower mortality. Furthermore, Kohout, et al. (2002) found a relationship between optimism and better immune functioning.

Other studies either failed to show a positive relationship between optimism and health in older adults or showed a negative relationship. For example, Schofield, et al. (2004) found no relationship between optimism and cancer survival, while Schulz, et al. (1996) failed to find a relationship between optimism and longevity. In fact, some studies (Segestrom, 2001) indicated that optimism was related to worse immune functioning.

Research on psychosocial stressors has been unclear regarding the impact on older adults, i.e., are older individuals more vulnerable to psychosocial stressors than younger people? Studies have shown that the immune systems of older adults are more vulnerable to stress. For example, two studies (Kiecolt-Glaser, et al., 2002 and Vitaliano, 1995) have demonstrated that those who are depressed have a reduced functioning of the immune system. However, other studies have shown less vulnerability in older adults compared to middle-aged adults. Johnson, et al. (2000) found that older adults experiencing a loss of a spouse had lower risks of mortality than middle-aged adults in the same situation. Furthermore, older adults appraised physical and/or psychological traumas as less stressful than younger adults (Park, et al., 2005).

Religion and spirituality and the relationship with quality of life have also been examined. A large number of studies have suggested that older people who are involved in religion tend to enjoy better mental health, as well as physical health, when compared to those who are not religious. Although there is often a decline in church attendance with aging (Koenig, et al., 2001), there is often an increase in the use of prayer and positive religious coping responses (Pargament, 1997). Involvement in a church, or synagogue, or other religious institution, may offer both emotional and other support to the elderly, which in turn may bolster the individual's health and well being (Cohen, 2004). Support may well extend beyond the sanctuary itself.

A number of investigators have also examined the role of forgiveness and its relationship to quality of life. Older adults who forgive others tend to have better mental health than individuals who have difficulty forgiving (Thoresen, et al., 2000). In another study, Krause and Ellison (2003) found that forgiving immediately had a positive impact on mental health. Worthington (2004) indicated that individuals who forgive more quickly have lower levels of negative emotions.

There may also be negative consequences of religious involvement. For example, there may be negative interactions with other congregants or spiritual leaders. Krause, et al. (1998) found that people may experience more symptoms of depression when they experience negative interaction in the church. Krause (2003) also suggested that individuals who have doubts about their faith are more likely to have increased symptoms of psychological distress.

CASE STUDIES

The following two case studies illustrate the decline in quality of life that may be experienced by older adults.

Case 1

Caroline is a 96-year-old Caucasian woman, widowed for almost 25 years. She had been a homemaker. She resided in her own domicile until three years ago, when due to ambulation problems, she reluctantly moved into a nursing home for primarily middle class and upper middle class individuals. She has her own apartment, but has meals in a dining room where residents are served three meals per day. She has two adult children in the area, numerous grandchildren as well as great-grandchildren. Few friends are still alive, but she has made several new friends since moving into the nursing home. In addition, she attends church each Sunday and has a number of friends and family members who attend church with her. She tends to go for outings (besides church) at least one time per week. These include shopping, plays, movies and eating at restaurants. She also watches T.V., reads, talks on the phone and to fellow residents, but rarely participates in activities sponsored by the nursing home.

Caroline has suffered from OP for over twenty years and takes medication daily. She has no other chronic ailments, but had experienced pulmonary function problems in the past. She also

CASE STUDIES—Cont'd

walks daily, although she now needs to utilize a walker. She is physically slim, perhaps somewhat below average in weight. She generally eats well, but no longer exercises except for limited walking. Cognitive faculties are excellent, although her short-term memory has decreased somewhat in an age-appropriate way. There is no evidence of depression or acute anxiety. However, she periodically expresses a desire that "God take me already."

Case 2

Morris is a 71-year-old Caucasian male, married for 45 years. He has three adult children, but only one lives in the area. He retired when he was 64 years old, selling his business. Morris resides with his wife in an upper middle class suburb in a large metropolitan city. He suffered a heart attack when he was 67 years old and subsequently had open-heart surgery. Following the surgery, he developed acute anxiety and later depression. He refused to leave the home, exercise (as requested by his physicians) and avoided friends. His wife became increasingly frustrated with him and his steadfast resistance to do anything. She began to see a psychologist herself, and eventually took him to a geriatric psychiatrist, who placed him on medication.

He continued to avoid friends and family, as well as activities. His physical condition deteriorated as well. He had several additional hospitalizations for cardiac problems. When his wife, who worked part-time, would go to work, he would have increased anxiety attacks. As a result, he was placed in an adult daycare facility when she was at work. However, he refused to participate in any activities or with other individuals, and resists even going to the facility. His depression has exacerbated and has not responded to treatment. Furthermore, he refuses to speak to a therapist, although family members have availed themselves of the geriatric psychiatrist's assistance. He has expressed angry feelings as well, to the point that family members have a tendency to avoid him. Morris consistently expresses a desire to "leave me alone."

4
Psychological Problems
in the Elderly

According to the White House Conference on Aging, mental illness is the leading threat to independence and quality of life in older adults. The prevalence of mental illness among nursing home residents has consistently been found to be high. Two-thirds of residents were found to have diagnosable mental disorders and one-fourth suffer from depression. However, some individuals appear to be at greater risk for developing depression and/or anxiety in later adulthood. Wilson, et al. (2006) found that childhood adversity was associated with less adaptive psychosocial functioning in old age. In particular, emotional neglect and parental intimidation during childhood had the highest associations with less adaptive emotional functioning in later life.

As individuals age, chronic illnesses increase significantly. Concomitantly, there is also an increase in psychological symptoms as well as emotional disorders. According to the Cleveland Clinic (2003), chronic illness may affect a person's mobility and independence, and effect the way a person lives, see him or herself and/or relates to others. There are often dramatic changes in psychological and social functioning. A certain amount of sadness is normal, but at times, chronic disease may result in depression, anxiety, anger, sleep disorders and/or substance abuse.

Multiple changes occur in the aging brain, leading to age-related emotional disorders. A growing body of recent evidence suggests that the cortical delta-opoid receptor system plays a critical role in anxiety and depressive-like behaviors. Narita, et al. (2006) found that the aging process promotes astrogliosis or an abnormal increase of astrocytes in the cingulated cortex, leading to emotional disorders. Blazer and Hybels (2005) found that older adults appear to be at greater risk for major depression biologically as a result of vascular changes. Yet, older adults may be protected psychologically due to factors such as socio-emotional selectivity and wisdom and be protected from social risks compared to younger adults.

The risk of getting depression is 10-25% for older women and 5-12% for older men, but it is much higher for older adults with chronic diseases, often 25-33%, according to the Cleveland Clinic (2003). The rate of depression for those with multiple sclerosis (MS) and Parkinson's disease was found to be 40%, while the rate of depression was even higher for those with coronary heart disease (CHD), who have had a heart attack. Forty to sixty-five percent of these individuals experience depression. Sullivan (1992) found that patients with chronic low back pain had a prevalence of major depression three to four times greater than the normal population.

In particular, chronic illnesses and aging have been associated with an increase in depressive symptoms and depressive disorders (Anderson, et al., 2001). Common symptoms of depression include: depressed mood, loss of energy, decreased motivation, loss of interest or pleasure in daily activities (adhedonia), problems with concentration, and/or problems with memory (particularly short term memory). There may also be sleep problems, loss of appetite, feelings of worthlessness, feelings of guilt, increased irritability, feelings of hopelessness, crying spells and recurrent thoughts of suicide or death.

At times, depression results from a specific biologic effect of a medical condition, as with multiple sclerosis (MS), Parkinson's disease and cerebrovascular disease. In other instances, behavioral mechanisms have a role, in that the individual has limitations placed upon the person; there is a gradual withdrawal from enjoyable activities (Prince, et al., 1998).

In a longitudinal study (van Gool, et al., 2005), the researchers discovered that depression significantly increased modified the associations between pathology and subsequent impairment. In addition, they found an accelerating effect of depression on disability. Yang (2005) found that both stable disability status and transitions in disability status were significantly related to change in depressive symptoms.

Onishi, et al. (2004) studied the etiology of depressive mood in older adults and found that depression was often associated with handicaps. In particular, the loss of hope and morale, as well as memory loss and reduction of physical activity were highly correlated with depression. Strawbridge, et al. (2002) discovered that greater physical activity was protective for both prevalent depression and incident depression. In another study, Ragland, et al. (2005) reported that increased depression might be among the consequences associated with driving reduction or cessation. Increased depression for former drivers was substantially higher in men than in women.

Research has also shown that each person is affected differently by disease and disability. Jang, et al. (2004) reported that there were age differences in older adult's perceptions of health and depressive symptoms. Individuals with advanced old age were less affected by disability in comparison to the younger group of elderly. In addition, the authors found that regardless of age, the effects of disease and disability were mediated through subjective health perceptions.

Psychosocial factors, especially depression, seem to impact the development and/or the progression of a number of chronic diseases such as CHD and diabetes mellitus (DM) (Schneiderman, et al., 2001). Frequently, patients as well as their families overlook the symptoms of depression, assuming that the depression is normal, but temporary for an individual coping with a serious, chronic disease. In addition, symptoms of depression are often masked by other medical conditions, which results in treatment of the symptoms but not the underlying cause of the depression. For example, some chronic illnesses such as Parkinson's disease and MS have both a biological and an environmental component to the depression, which only serves to further complicate the diagnosis and subsequent treatment. In one study of Puerto Rican elderly (Robison, et al., 2003), the findings indicated that social stressors and inadequate support substantially increased the risk of depression. Those with the lowest income, more recent migration and poor subjective health were significantly more likely to be depressed. In addition, those who saw few relatives each month, those with family and/or financial problems and those caring for grandchildren also had significantly higher rates of depression.

Depression also exacerbates the impact of chronic illness. Studies have shown an association between depression and mortality resulting from cardiovascular disease (Unutzer, et al., 2002). Marzari, et al. (2005) reported that depressive symptomatology conferred an increased risk for CHD in men and for mortality in men and women. Glassman, et al. (1998) found an association between depression and ischemic heart disease. However, researchers in

Holland (Licht-Strunk, et al., 2004) related that there was no evidence to support the hypothesis that depressed older persons with vascular disease, have a distinct depressive symptom profile.

In another study, de Groot, et al. (2001) reported that depression was connected with a poorer prognosis and more rapid progression of chronic illnesses, including diabetes. Anderson, et al. (2001) studied patients with Type 1 and Type 2 DM and reviewed 39 studies. They related that DM doubled the chances of developing depression. In addition, the authors concluded that the odds of depression were significantly higher in women than in men. This finding mirrored the female preponderance of depression in epidemiological studies of the general population. In another study (Gavard, et al., 1993), depression was discovered to exist in 14.7% and elevated depression symptoms in 26% of diabetic patients.

Although there have been a number of studies on depression with older adults, there has been much less research on suicide in the elderly. The rate of completed suicide has been found to be elevated relative to the general population, particularly in those suffering from chronic illnesses (Fisher, et al., 2001). The literature on suicide suggests that chronic pain patients, particularly those who are elderly, are at greater risk for depression than the general population. Fishbain (1999) reviewed 18 studies relating to the association of suicide and chronic pain and found that suicide ideation, suicide attempts and gestures as well as successful suicide were commonly found in patients with chronic pain. Not surprisingly, a high percentage of these individuals were elderly. In addition, in a number of studies, chronic pain was postulated to be a suicide risk factor.

DeLeo and Spathonis (2003) reviewed epidemiological studies of suicide in the elderly and discovered that assisted suicide and euthanasia in older adults were associated with the desire to escape chronic physical pain and suffering caused by illness, as well as to relieve the psychological pain and feelings of hopelessness and depression. In another study, Gonzales (1995) found that the risk of suicide was significantly greater in patients with poorly controlled pain. Furthermore, Penttinen (1995) found a relationship between back pain and suicide in Finnish farmers. Mellick, et al. (1992) found that degenerative illness and pain were both risk factors in suicide. Fishbain (1991) studied patients in a pain center and reported that the completed suicide rate was significantly higher for chronic pain patients than that of the general population.

In another study, Stenager, et al. (1994) found that among those who attempted suicide, 52% suffered from a disease and 21% were on daily analgesics. Smith, et al. (2004) discovered that chronic pain patients with self-reported insomnia and high pain intensity were more likely to report passive suicidal ideation. Roscoe, et al. (2003) found that poorly controlled pain was a factor in seeking assistance in dying. In this study, the patients of Dr. Jack Kevorkian were studied; the most common diagnoses were amyotrophic lateral sclerosis or MS, inadequately controlled pain and a recent decline in health. Emanuel, et al. (1996) related that oncology patients with concomitant pain and depression were significantly more likely to request assistance in suiciding, as well as actively taking steps to end their own lives. In another study, Macfarlane, et al. (2001) reported that there were higher mortality rates in patients with widespread body pain, including patients with fibromyalgia. Finally, Magni, et al. (1998) found that those with chronic pain had suicide attempts, suicidal thoughts and thoughts about death two to three times greater than those without chronic pain.

Although depression is clearly the most common psychological disorder and symptom reported by the elderly, many individuals also report anxiety symptoms as well. In one study (de Beurs, et al., 2005), self reported self report data taken from the Longitudinal Aging Study in Amsterdam were used and the investigators reported that there was an association between low mastery, high neuroticism and an increase in negative affect, lack of positive affect and anxiety. Brenes, et al. (2005) discovered that anxiety was a significant risk factor for the progression of disability in older women. In another study, Torras-Garcia, et al. (2005) postulated that aging may lead to decreased levels of anxiety.

Other studies have focused on the relationship between pain and anxiety. Hadjistavropoulos, et al. (2002) reported that health anxiety played a role in pain behavior. However, other studies have found a high degree of variability in anxiety among individuals with chronic pain. Nonetheless, increased anxiety may contribute to sleep disturbance and/or insomnia. In particular, those individuals with anxiety, depression and chronic pain may suffer from sleep disturbance, which in turn has a role in increased anxiety and depression. Furthermore, difficulty with sleep can also exacerbate stress and/or make it more difficult to cope with stress.

There has also been considerable research on alcohol problems in older adults. Interestingly, there is ample evidence that health care providers across the spectrum of primary, acute and long-term care providers ignore the signs and symptoms of alcohol abuse and dependence in the elderly rather than confronting the problem. Stevenson (2005) has noted that older alcohol misusers and abusers are at excess risk for a myriad of physical problems and premature death, because alcohol negatively interacts with some drugs and the natural aging process, thus increasing the risk for injuries, hypertension, cardiac problems, cancers, gastrointestinal problems, bone loss and neurocognitive problems. Furthermore, the abuse of alcohol has a strong association with depression in both the general population and more specifically in the elderly. Research has shown that higher levels of alcohol contribute to bone loss and falls, blood clots in the coronary and brain vessels and cognitive decline.

While it is often thought that alcohol consumption decreases with age, the VA Normative Aging Study (Levinson, et al., 1998) revealed a more complex picture. While fewer older men drink, often due to negative interactions with medications, those who continued to drink did so at levels consistent with past alcohol use. In another study, Moos, et al. (2004) found evidence of decreased alcohol use in older adults who continued to drink.

Although alcohol or other drugs may assist an elderly person in falling to sleep, in fact, alcohol and many other drugs, including marijuana, interferes with adequate sleep and particularly with REM sleep. In turn, a vicious cycle is created, with the individual then increasingly relying on the drug to help deal with insomnia. This is particularly true with individuals with chronic pain and/or depression, where self-medication may be a means of coping. Johnson (1996) reported that elderly women were at high risk for abusing alcohol and psychotropic medications in their attempt to control pain and ameliorate sleep problems.

Personality changes associated with aging have been debated for numerous years. Freud believed that personality development was relatively complete by the time an individual reached adolescence and that little change was possible after age 40. However, Jung disagreed and argued that personality develops throughout one's life in response to changing life experiences. Some longitudinal studies revealed that basic personality traits remained generally stable over an adult's life, including traits such as neuroticism and extroversion, while other studies have shown changes in other aspects of personality, particularly an increased preoccupation with one's inner life (Caspi and Roberts, 2001; Costa and McRae, 1994; and Roberts and Delvecchio, 2000). More recently, it has been postulated that individual differences are variable and that some people are stable and some are not stable.

Studies showing individual differences in the rate of change in personality traits are plentiful (Helson, et al., 2002; Jones, et al., 2003; Small, et al., 2003). Even though it is fairly clear that some people change more than others, it is far less clear why some individuals remain stable and others change. Studies have examined the impact of the environment, genetic makeup and how proactive one is in changing. Studies have also been conducted to assess the relationship between personality and mortality. Friedman, et al. (1993) assessed personality from childhood and found that greater impulsiveness was associated with earlier death and that conscientiousness was related to better health outcomes. Wilson, et al. (2004) found that this relationship between conscientiousness and longer life held for older adults as well.

Changes in personality accompany forms of slow-moving but debilitating neurological disorders, including Alzheimer's disease (AD) and mini strokes. A number of researchers, particularly Berg (1996); Small and Backman (1997); and Small, et al. (2003) have attributed "terminal decline" to neurological problems and Berg (1996) has indicated that this may also be related to personality.

CASE STUDIES

The following three case studies show some of the different ways in which older adults may respond to stressors in their lives.

Case 1

Molly is an 81 year-old Caucasian woman, widowed three years ago. She had been a teacher for over 30 years until retiring 9 years ago. She continues to reside in her own residence and is active in her church and charities. Since her husband's death, she has traveled extensively, visiting her four children and their families and also going on several elder hostel learning trips. She has an active network of friends, primarily through her church.

CASE STUDIES—Cont'd

She exercises daily and plays bridge, both at the senior center in her community. She also reads for at least one-hour per day, and regularly attends plays, the ballet, the symphony and movies. She does not smoke but drinks one glass of wine two to three times per week. Molly displays no signs of depression, anxiety or any other psychological disorder. Her health is still excellent, although she has had surgery to remove polyps in her colon on threeoccasions.

Case 2

Sandra is a 76 year old Hispanic woman, married for 56 years. She had been a homemaker her entire life and has only worked part-time at a retail store during the Christmas holidays when she was younger. She has five children. Three of the children live out of state, while two children and their families live in the area. Her husband, Julio, has had AD for the past four years. At this point, he may not always recognize her. She has insisted in caring for Julio at home and has refused help except from one daughter, who comes over two times per week to help. Since the diagnosis, she has become increasingly depressed. She sleeps fitfully, and suffers from middle sleep disorder, usually waking up one or two times per night and laying awake for at least one-hour each time. Although she always drank one or two cocktails each night with her husband throughout her marriage, her drinking has increased substantially in the past three years. At the present time, she typically drinks between a pint and a quart of vodka daily, usually "passing out" on the couch. On several occasions she has fallen down, one time falling down the stairs to the basement and severely bruising herself. She continues to attend church regularly, but no longer participates in social activities through the church or with friends. When old friends call, she makes excuses as to why she cannot see them. She has also made excuses as to why friends may not come to the home, typically indicating that Julio becomes upset with changes in routine.

Several of her children have suggested that she see her doctor for medication for depression, but she refuses to do so. Her daughter has also expressed concerns about her mother's physical condition, in that Sandra is at least 50 pounds overweight and primarily eats fried food. Her children have no knowledge of her increased use of alcohol, although her daughter suspects there may be a problem.

Case 3

William is a 62 year old Caucasian male, married for 29 years. He has two adolescent children. He grew up in an abusive home environment, with an alcoholic father. William had been a captain in a local fire department until four years ago, when he was diagnosed with MS. Since the diagnosis, he has been on disability. Initially, he attempted to remain active, insisting on walking himself, even though this resulted in numerous falls. Eventually, he had to resort to a walker and later a wheel chair.

As his disease progressed, he became increasingly angry, often yelling at his wife and children, as well as close friends. Frustration tolerance was low and irritability was high. In addition, he became significantly depressed, marked by decreased appetite, poor concentration, decreased memory, low energy, adhedonia, feelings of hopelessness, minimal motivation, as well as suicidal thoughts and ideation. He was referred to a psychiatrist and started on anti-depressant medication. He refused to see a counselor. However, his wife and children began therapy to assist them in coping with William, and in dealing with their own anger towards him.

As William lost further muscle control, he became even more angry and depressed. He began to spend his days watching TV in bed and withdrew from all contact with friends. He refused to leave the home, even when invited by extended family or friends. As his depression worsened, he made a suicide attempt, ingesting pills and was rushed to the hospital. A consulting psychiatrist met with him, but to no avail. He again refused to see a therapist and also refused occupational therapy and/or physical therapy.

5
Cognitive Changes in Older Adults

As people age, they undergo a number of physiological changes, involving a general slowing down of all organ systems due to a gradual decline in cellular activity. For some, the level of decline may be dramatic and rapid while for others the changes are slow and seem insignificant. In spite of anatomical and physiological declines, numerous research studies have found only limited decrements in actual intellectual functioning associated with the aging process. Most older adults experience virtually no functional impairment despite their cognitive limitations. In fact, the current research on aging indicates that cognitive decline is not an inevitable function of the aging process. Moreover, individuals can take steps to maintain cognitive health throughout life. Butler, et al. (2004) reported that social engagement, intellectual stimulation and physical activity play significant roles in maintaining cognitive health and preventing cognitive decline. Other researchers (Anstey and Low, 2004) have noted that many of the risk factors for cognitive aging are modifiable. These include diabetes, hypertension and levels of social, mental and physical activity.

Speed of Processing

Fluid abilities including speed and problem solving decline with normal aging (Anstey and Low, 2004). On intelligence tests, a classic aging pattern involving poorer performance on tests of fluid intelligence has been consistently demonstrated. Some of the earliest research on age-related behavioral decline proposed that the decline was the result of fundamental changes in the central nervous system (Birren, 1974; Birren and Renner, 1977). These authors suggested that the slowing might be the result of degenerative change in the basal ganglia. Graybiel (2000) noted that the basal ganglia are richly connected in feedback-feed forward circuits with large parts of the cortex. LaBerge (1995) cited the role of the thalmi in a similar vein. These circuits serve to select some stimuli for processing while suppressing others. In addition, these circuits select some lines of activity to be stimulated and other lines to be inhibited. Damage and/or dysfunction in these circuits, could potentially affect most, if not all, cortical functioning.

The fact that older persons seem to perform more poorly on tests of fluid intelligence is due in part to reduced efficiency of nerve transmission in the brain, resulting in slower information processing and greater loss of information during transmission. However, performance decrements may also be due to a variety of non-cognitive factors, including impairments in sensation and/or motor ability. The older adult's slower motor performance can significantly impact the ability to respond on tests that require fine hand movements, i.e., filling in the proper circles on an answer sheet. Sensory deficits associated with aging may result in perceptual inaccuracies, requiring more attention and cognitive effort to recognizing sensory input thus, reducing the brain's capacity to quickly process new information.

When older adults make decisions, they have been found to sacrifice speed for accuracy, for they tend to work slowly, examining the pros and cons of issues before selecting a response. In addition, even when cognitive competencies are affected by the aging process, older adults have been found to develop compensating strategies. For example, older typists have been found to type as quickly and as accurately as younger typists even though they are unable to move their fingers as fast. They have developed a better ability to anticipate upcoming words and locate the proper keys.

Salthouse (1985) reported that the correlation between chronological age and reaction time averaged .45 in 39 separate studies. This implies that 20% of the variance in reaction time is attributed to age. However, Salthouse noted that older adults might be less practiced at the tasks utilized to measure reaction time. In addition, some authors (Clarkson-Smith and Hartley (1989, 1990) demonstrated that age-related differences can be lowered in aerobically conditioned older people and in athletes. However, the vast majority of research has clearly shown that latencies and slower speed of responses is characteristic of aging. In fact, Cerella (1990) indicated that there were systematic relationships between the reaction times of younger adults and those of older adults across a range of tasks. Other researchers (Fisher and Glaser, 1996; Ratcliff, et al., 2000, 2004) have generally agreed with Cerella's hypothesis, but have expanded the original research.

In more recent research, Rabbitt, et al. (2004) suggested that slowing down is simply a marker or a correlate of other changes. They commented that reaction time may reflect the general intactness of the nervous system, by reflecting the accumulated effect of numerous small and disparate age-related changes, because responses in most speed tasks require a number of operations performed under time pressure. Furthermore, Salthouse and Caja (2000) have posited that the underlying cause for age-related differences is a general reduction in functional intactness of the central nervous system.

Several researchers (Christensen, et al., 2001; Salthouse, 1998, 2001) have related that the association between speed or sensory acuity and cognitive variables might simply be an artifact of the relationship each of these factors has with age. Christensen, et al. (2001) studied 374 Australian subjects in four age ranges and measured several factors including reaction time, recall, recognition, abstract thinking and vocabulary. Demographic factors, such as gender and education were also evaluated. There were direct effects of age on fluid intellectual factors. In another study, Salthouse and Ferrer-Caja (2003) studied 204 people from age 20 to 91. Scores for speed and processing memory declined significantly with increasing age.

Anstey, et al. (2003) collected data from 1823 people from the Australian Longitudinal Study of Aging. Measures of cognitive performance included verbal ability, memory, processing speed, visual acuity and auditory acuity. The preliminary findings indicated that the factor structure for the cognitive and sensory latent variables was stable over time. However, their data also suggested that there appear to be independent processes that affect some abilities but not others.

Braver, et al. (2001) posited that the gradual loss of the ability to gather and use contextual clues could explain the age related cognitive decline across a variety of functions. The authors suggest that erratic or declining dopamine levels may have a broad impact on the skills of attention, inhibition, and episodic and working memory involved in context processing. Braver, et al. (2001) compared the performance of 175 young adults and 81 older adults on an AX Continuous Performance Test and measured how quickly and accurately participants hit a button when they saw an "X" on a computer screen. The researchers found that older adults performed worse when contextual processing was assessed, and that under conditions of interference, age-related differences were accentuated. Significantly, older adults had "fewer false alarms" because their impaired context processing slowed down their responses.

Memory

Most persons experience a modest increase in memory problems as they age, particularly with regard to the ability to remember relatively recent experiences. Decrements have been found both in the ability to accumulate new information and in the ability to retrieve existing information from memory storage, although there is little decline in the ability to store new information once it is learned. Mild memory impairment was found in 28% of a sample of healthy older adults in the community (Weaver Cargin, et al., 2006). African American older adults have been shown to perform poorer in terms of memory self-efficacy and memory performance (McDougall, 2004).

The process of learning new information and encoding it for storage requires more time as individuals age, because of the reduced efficiency of neural transmission and because of sensory deficits that limit one's ability to quickly and accurately perceive information to be learned. As a result, this may prevent individual experiences from being completely encoded into secondary memory. In addition, the accumulation of life experiences makes it more likely that new information may be inadequately distinguished from previous learning, thus making it difficult to establish unique cues and linkages for the new experiences.

As people age, they experience a decline in their ability to retrieve stored information. In part, this is due to the difficulty in extracting the correct bit of information from the from the lifetime accumulation of experiences. This can be particularly hard when the new information resembles previously learned information, such as when one is attempting to recall one phone number from all of the phone numbers resident in the memory. Therefore, it is not surprising that older adults do worse than their younger counterparts on tests of free recall, where they are asked to retrieve learned information but only given minimal cues. Yet, older adults are found to perform significantly better when given sufficient orienting parameters to limit the scope of the search or are asked to select the correct answer from a limited number of options, for example on a true-false or multiple choice test.

Older adults have more difficulty than younger people in tasks that involve episodic memory, that is, tasks that involve conscious retrieval of specific events located in time and place and/or retrieval of the context of experienced events. Episodic memory relies largely on recollection (Li, et al., 2004; Mark and Rugg, 1998). As people age, their performance in tasks that tap the conscious collection of prior experiences declines substantially with age (Blackman, et al., 2001; Light, et al., 2000; Zacks, et al., 2000). Age-related deficits in episodic memory have been found to reflect weakly formed associations at encoding, also known as blinding deficits (Li, et al., 2005; Naveh-Benjamin, 2000). Others have posited that these deficits are the result of the demands of attention at either encoding or retrieval (Castel and Craik, 2003; Naveh-Benjamin, 2001; Naveh-Benjamin et al., 2005).

Dixon, et al. (2004) assembled two different longitudinal samples of normal older adults, using a large battery of episodic memory indicators. Overall, an examination of performance on sets of common and complementary episodic tasks revealed that the changes over three years were modest. When decline occurred, it was gradual.

Older adults also show deficits in remembering source information (Spencer and Raz, 1995). Age-related deficits of source memory, as well as episodic memory, probably involve the failure to adequately associate target items with other items or target items with their contexts (Chalfonte and Johnson, 1996; Naveh-Benjamin, 2000; Naveh-Benjamin, et al., 2003, 2004). Several MRI and PET studies have demonstrated the role of the left prefrontal cortex and the hippocampus in age-related associative deficits in source memory (Mitchell, et al., 2000).

There has been considerable research on age differences in the susceptibility to false memory, and its relationship to deficits in source memory as well as episodic memory. Jacoby, et al. (2005) related that older adults were substantially more vulnerable to interference effects. They found that older adults were ten times more likely to falsely remember misleading information than younger adults. It is likely that an impoverished memory for the details of actual events renders the elderly more vulnerable than younger people to falsely accepting misinformation, accounting for the large number of older adults who fall prey to con-artists and scams.

Working memory has also been shown to decline with age. Working memory is involved in tasks that necessitate the individual simultaneously storing and actively transforming information. The greatest deficits in working memory occur in tasks such as reading span, listening span and operation span (Bopp and Verhaeghen, 2005; Verhaeghen and Salthouse, 1997). Large age differences were also demonstrated in several other laboratory studies (Byrne, 1998; Oberauer and Kliegl, 2001; Oberauer, et al., 2003; Reuter-Lorenz and Sylvester, 2005; Zelinski and Burnight, 1997). By contrast, relatively small age differences have been found in short-duration memory tasks that do not require much controlled or concurrent processing. This would include tasks such as digit span.

Mattay, et al. (2006) studied the neurophysiological correlates of age-related reduction in working memory capacity in younger and older subjects and showed that compensatory mechanisms such as additional prefrontal cortical activity are called upon to maintain efficiency in task performance. Older subjects had longer reaction times than their younger counterparts at all levels of task difficulty. Furthermore, at higher working memory loads, older adults performed worse than younger subjects. In another study, Duverne, et al. (2006) researched whether working memory executive components mediated the effects of age on strategy selection or strategy execution. They concluded that strategy selection changes with age. Older adults mainly selected one type of strategy while younger adults selected several types of strategies. In addition, strategy execution also changed with age, as demonstrated by agerelated differences on the hardest problems.

Significant relationships have also been shown between short-term memory capacity and fluid intelligence, as well as between working memory capacity and fluid intelligence. There has also been data demonstrating a relationship between working memory and spatial and language abilities (Kemper, et al., 2003; Kyllonen, 1996). Furthermore, Fabiani, et al. (2006) suggested that age-related changes in sensory processing are likely due to inefficient filtering of repeated information, rather than due to faster memory decay.

Stern, et al. (2005) explored the relationship between subjects' network expression during the performance of a memory test and an index of cognitive reserve. Older adults with higher cognitive reserve showed decreased expression of functionally connected regions of the brain. This suggests that for older subjects the set of functionally connected regions may represent an altered, compensatory network that is used to maintain function as age related physiological changes occur. Yamamoto and Shimada (2006) examined the cognitive aging mechanism of signaling effects on the memory for procedural sentences. Results indicated that signaling supported changes in strategy utilization during the successive organizational processes, and changes in strategy utilization resulting from signaling improved memory for procedural sentences. It was also shown that age-related factors interfered with these signaling effects.

Prospective memory, which refers to an individual's intentions for actions to be carried out in the future, has been found to be less effected by age than many other forms of memory, including episodic memory (Henry, et al., 2004). This has been shown to be true whether the task is time based (for example remembering to do a task at a certain time) or event based (for example remembering to do a task when a particular event occurs). Differences in performance in event based tasks have been shown to be greater when the demands on prospective memory are higher. This would include tasks when the association between cue and action is weak, tasks when cues are not especially relevant and tasks when the embedded task is highly engaging. However, older adults consistently outperform their younger counterparts in naturalistic prospective studies, for example when they are asked to telephone at specified times or asked to mail back postcards at certain times. It has been postulated that older adults may utilize effective external devices, perhaps as the result of years of experience with their declining episodic memory.

Learning

Research suggests that with the aging of the population, the number of persons with cognitive impairment is likely to increase. Comijs, et al. (2005) collected data from 1,349 older adults in the Longitudinal Aging Study Amsterdam and found cognitive decline and changes in cognitive functioning in older persons who were either not impaired or only mildly impaired at the beginning of the study. McGuire, et al. (2006) examined the impact of cognitive functioning on functional disability and mortality and showed that persons with lower levels of cognitive functioning were more likely to become disabled or die than those with higher levels of cognitive functioning. Other research has demonstrated that older adults experience a progressive decline in neuropsychological tasks requiring flexible adaptation to external feedback, which could be related to impairments in reward association learning. Mell, et al. (2005) posited that structural alterations of reward detecting structures and functional changes of the dopaminergic, as well as the serotonergic system might contribute to deficits in reward association learning. However, Mackinnon, et al. (2006) found that there was not support for the existence of developmental changes in the structure of cognitive and biological variables across the lifespan. Other studies (Helmes, et al., 2006) have attempted to assess whether there are gender differences in cognitive functioning with age; the results have not shown significance.

Dennis, et al. (2006) compared young and older adults on serial response time tasks in an effort to assess implicit sequence learning. Their results indicated that both younger and older adults were able to learn purely perceptual auditory sequences, but that explicit knowledge contributes to learning of sequences by young adults. Lien, et al. (2006) examined the automaticity of word recognition and concluded that greater cumulative experience with lexical processing leads to increased automaticity, allowing older adults to more efficiently perform. In another study, Pluchon, et al. (2002) demonstrated that normal aging corresponds with rising difficulties to name faces. However, they also showed that recognition of faces tends to be better preserved and that the greater weakness in recalling a name is linked to difficulties in lexical accessing. In another study, Phillips and Allen (2004) found that older adults perceived lower levels of emotional intensity in sad and happy faces, perhaps reflecting due to lower levels of anxiety and depression and better emotional adjustment with older age.

It has also been shown that aging is associated with declines in automatic processing of time-dependent stimulus features and that this is related to cognitive function. There are age-related declines in prefrontal cortex function and associated increases in susceptibility to task-irrelevant stimuli. Kisley and his colleagues

(2005) studied the effect of age on automatic processing on time-dependent stimulus features by measuring the auditory mismatch negativity (MMN) in younger and older adults and found that older adults demonstrated a decline on neuropsychological tests.

Schneider, et al. (2005) reported that speech comprehension declines more rapidly in older adults than in younger adults as speech rate increases. This effect had been attributed to a slowing of brain function with age. However, Schneider and his colleagues suggested that auditory decline rather than cognitive slowing may be responsible for older adults' decreased performance in speeded conditions. Valentijn, et al. (2005) examined the longitudinal relationship between sensory functioning and a broad range of cognitive functions after 6-year follow-up and whether cataract surgery or first-time hearing aid use affected cognition. Their findings supported a connection between sensory acuity in both the auditory and visual domains and cognitive measures, both from a cross sectional and longitudinal perspective.

Maurits, et al. (2006) investigated changes in coherence with aging during cognitive tasks. Their results indicated that aging is associated with increased EEG coherence during a relatively easy cognitive task. Previously, several MRI and PET studies of cognitive tasks found increased bilateral activity in elderly subjects. Saykin, et al. (2006) utilized MRI scans and found that older adults with cognitive complaints had neurodegenerative changes on MRI scans, not yet evident on neuropsychological evaluation. Specifically, there was decreased gray matter, with differences evident in the medial temporal lobe, frontotemporal and other neocortical regions. Thomas, et al. (2004) examined aging and cognition utilizing CT scan and found that age related changes of the white matter were associated with a decreased cognitive state. Grady, et al. (2006) used MRI to examine brain activity during encoding and recognition tasks and found that there was a gradual, age-related reduction in the ability to suspend non-task related or "default mode" activity and engage areas for carrying out memory tasks. Dennis, et al. (2006) also utilized MRI examinations in studying encoding.

Their results showed age-related reductions in the left hippocampus, but increases in the left prefrontal cortex. Huh, et al. (2006) found a relationship between frontal regions and response bias (the decision rule an individual uses when faced with uncertainty on recognition memory tasks).

Effects of Disease

Much of the research on the effect of disease on cognitive functioning has focused on Alzheimer's disease (AD), which is the most common cause of dementia in older adults. A number of authors, including Cole and Tak (2006) have indicated that impaired memory is characteristic of AD. According to Hedden and Gabrieli (2005), AD is characterized by severe hippocampal injury, although early-stage AD may relatively spare some cortical regions. Golby, et al. (2005) found that MRI findings revealed impairment in the mesial temporal lobe and fusiform regions, suggesting dissociation in AD between impaired explicit memory encoding in the mesial temporal lobe and fusiform regions. In another study, Fleischman, et al. (2005) found that the hallmark indices of AD are associated with performance on priming tests to the extent that conceptual, but not perceptual, processing resources are required. Higher levels of AD pathology was related to lower levels of explicit memory. Bucks and Radford (2004) found a significant difference between a healthy adult group and an AD group on cognition tasks, as well as on emotion tasks.

Studies on dementia have consistently shown that individuals with dementia overestimate their cognitive and functional abilities. However, Farias, et al. (2005) demonstrated that individuals with mild cognitive impairment do not appear to under-report their functioning. By contrast, those with AD have been found to not recognize cognitive deficits and to experience anosognosia (unawareness of disease). Those with frontotemporal dementia have been shown to experience a loss of insight. A study by Rankin, et al. (2005) demonstrated differences between those with AD, those with frontotemporal dementia and normal older adults. The group with frontotemporal dementia showed the greatest magnitude of error in the largest number of personality dimensions and tended to exaggerate positive qualities and minimize negative qualities, more than those with AD.

The impact of other diseases on cognition has been studied, but to a lesser degree than research on AD and dementia. Louis, et al. (2005) examined patients with Parkinsonian signs and found that mild Parkinsonian signs, especially rigidity, were associated with mild cognitive impairment. Mackowiak-Cordoliani, et al. (2005) reported that there was an increased risk of dementia after stroke. In another study, de Mendonca, et al. (2005) found the presence of sub cortical vascular disease was common in older adults with mild cognitive impairment, but does not appear to be associated with the severity of cognitive deficits. Prins, et al. (2005) found that cerebral small-vessel disease may contribute to cognitive decline in older adults by affecting information processing speed and executive function. Stern, et al. (2004) found a relationship between mild alterations of thyroid hormone levels and changes in cognitive functioning and mood in older adults.

There has also been research on the association between prescription medication and changes in cognitive functioning across the life span. Starr, et al. (2004) reported that the degree to which drugs impair cognition in relatively healthy, older people may not be apparent. However, their results indicated that statins, often used for cardiovascular disease, may be promising in ameliorating cognitive decline in older people.

CASE STUDIES

The following two cases reflect the impact of non-problematic cognitive aging and early stage AD.

Case 1

John is a 73 year old Caucasian male, widowed eight years ago. He had been a school superintendent for 24 years before he retired 7 years ago. John has numerous hobbies, including investments, swimming, golfing, tennis and bridge. He attends church regularly and is involved in several committees through his church, including chairman of the new members committee. He has lunch with various friends several days per week and belongs to a country club and plays golf, tennis and bridge there several days per week. He has two female friends and "dates" both. John has three children, one who lives in his area. He sees this daughter and her family on a weekly basis. He visits his other two children and their families at least four times per year. Although John suffered a stroke approximately two years ago, he worked hard in his rehab program and follows a strict regimen of exercise, diet and medication. At times, he acknowledges feeling "down," but enjoys life for the most part. He gets frustrated when he cannot recall someone's name or a phone number, but accepts his limitations.

Case 2

Margaret is an 80 year old African American female, widowed 15 years ago. She had worked as an administrative assistant for the same company for over forty years prior to retirement 15 years ago. She has four children, all who reside in her city. She has weekly contact with all of them and often has babysat for various relatives. Margaret attends church several times per week and has a strong group of friends through church. She has no hobbies. Margaret was diagnosed with AD approximately two years ago and has a slow but steady decline in cognitive functioning. Initially, she had difficulty with short-term memory. More recently, she has experienced increasing problems with judgment, for example dressing inappropriately for the weather and/or situation. Her children have expressed a desire to have her live in a skilled-care facility, but she has insisted on living at home. A social worker has met with Margaret, but to no avail. In fact, she became very angry and "threw" the social worker out of her home. Margaret has also had a number of medical problems recently, primarily cardiovascular, and she has been inconsistent in taking medication.

6
Seniors with Diabetes Mellitus

As one ages, the ability of pancreatic beta-cells to react to glucose is reduced. (Thearle and Brillantes, 2005). This decline in beta-cell insulin secretion is a major factor in the development of diabetes mellitus (DM). Seniors with DM suffer higher rates of premature death, disability, and co-morbid health problems, including hypertension, coronary heart disease (CHD), and stroke than those without DM (California Healthcare Foundation/American Geriatrics Society Panel on Improving Care of Elders with Diabetes, 2003).

People over the age of 40, who have DM, are at risk of developing neuropathies, a family of nerve disorders associated with DM (National Diabetes Information Clearinghouse, 2002). Neuropathies result in numbness, pain, and weakness in the extremities. They may also affect other organ systems including the digestive system, heart, and sex organs. Symptoms include indigestion, nausea, or vomiting, diarrhea or constipation, problems with urination, and erectile dysfunction. The highest rates of neuropathy occur among people who have had DM for a minimum of 25 years. Other risk factors for diabetic neuropathy include difficulties controlling blood glucose levels, high levels of blood fat, hypertension, and being overweight and obese. Peripheral neuropathy, the most common type, affects the upper and lower extremities. Autonomic neuropathy, still another type, causes alterations in the digestive system, bladder function, sexual functioning, and perspiration.

Elder diabetics are at higher risk for developing geriatric syndromes, such as depression, cognitive dysfunction, urinary incontinence, injurious falls, and chronic pain, than non-diabetic older persons.

In addition, aged adults with DM may face a number of social and psychological problems. The assessment and treatment of this population should be cautiously customized based on their level of functioning, co-morbid health problems, as well as their lifestyle and life expectancy (Smitz, 2005; California Healthcare Foundation/American Geriatrics Society Panel on Improving Care of Elders with Diabetes, 2003; Rosenstock, 2001).

Complications and Risk Factors

In a Swedish study of 6-year mortality in elderly men and women living at home, Gustafsson, et al. (1998) showed that DM, heart problems, and overall self-ratings of poor health were independent predictors of mortality.

Elder diabetics who suffer diabetes-related complications have a higher mortality rate than older diabetics without complications (Otiniano, et al., 2003a). These complications include eye problems, kidney disease, lower extremity disease, chronic pain, and depression.

Racial/Ethnic and Socioeconomic Status Factors

Racial/ethnic, cultural and socioeconomic status factors have been found to be linked to diabetic complications.

Since members of ethnic and racial minorities have worse glycemic control than whites, they may be at higher risk for developing diabetic complications than whites. Using data from a cohort of 468 diabetics from the Health, Aging, and Body Composition Study, de Rekeneire, et al. (2003) discovered that blacks had poorer glycemic control than whites. These findings remained after adjusting for possible confounding factors. The study results also showed that differences in glycemic control predicted severity of the disease, health status, lower quality of care, but these factors did not fully account for the higher HbA1c levels in older black diabetics.

Aged Mexican-American and African-American diabetics may be especially vulnerable to DM complications such as cardiovascular disease, eye problems, kidney disease, circulation problems, and amputations. Drawing on data from the Hispanic Established Population for the Epidemiological Study of the Elderly (EPESE), Otiniano, et al. (2003a) discovered that the risk of 7-year mortality among Mexican-American elders increased with the number of diabetic complications. They found that patients with only one diabetic complication did not differ significantly in their 7-year mortality from the control group, but patients who suffered two or three diabetic complications were almost twice as likely to die within a seven year period when compared to those without any diabetic complications. Those patients with four diabetic complications were almost three times more likely to die within 7 years.

Gender and Diabetic Complications

Gender differences have been found for different types of diabetic complications. Based on random samples of 121 men and 223 women, ages 60 years and older and 93 men and 180 women ages, 35 to 59 years, Lerman, et al. (1998) found that more older Mexican men had diabetes mellitus than the women did.

Using data on diabetic Mexican-American elders, Otiniano, et al. (2003b) reported that more females than males had a lower extremity amputation at the start of their study.

Another investigation by Crooks, et al. (2003) evaluated the association between DM and cognitive performance in 3,681 women, aged 75 and older, and found that diabetic women had lower cognitive functioning than non-diabetic women.

Wachtel (2005) evaluated the association between family poverty and risk of diabetic complications among minorities, aged 50 years and older, and showed that family poverty predicted differences in diabetic amputation rates among African-Americans, Hispanic-Americans, and other individuals.

One investigation of Mexican-American diabetics, aged 65 and older, found that persons with less than 12 years of education had a greater chance of developing DM-related complications than those with less than 12 years of education (Otiniano, et al., 2002).

Hyperglycemia

Blaum, et al. (2005) used a random sample of 576 disabled women, aged 65 to 101 years, to determine whether cardiovascular disease, co-morbid health problems, and degree of hyperglycemia influenced DM-associated mortality risk. The results showed that disabled older women with DM had an increased risk for non-cardiovascular death, but not for cardiovascular death. The findings also indicated that among this population, mild, moderate, or severe hyperglycemia predicted an increased risk of mortality. The researchers concluded that vascular complications did not completely account for the total mortality risk.

Hypoglycemia

A major issue for clinicians is achieving appropriate glycemic goals for older diabetics while avoiding hypoglycemia (Chelliah and Burge, 2004). Older patients with DM are especially predisposed to hypoglycemia (Holstein and Egberts, 2003). They can suffer intense emotional distress from repeated episodes of hypoglycemia even when the episodes are fairly mild. In addition, hypoglycemia among in this population has been associated with increased health care costs.

Diabetic seniors are especially vulnerable to social isolation, depression, or illness, conditions, which can cause nutritional deficiencies and irregular self-monitoring of blood glucose levels. These problems can result in hypoglycemic episodes that, in turn may lead to changes in personality, a disabling fall, or other accident (PDRHealth, 2004).

Family members and friends often are unaware of the relationship between behavioral difficulties and hypoglycemic episodes. As a result, aged diabetics may be misdiagnosed as having dementia when, in reality, their symptoms are the result of missing meals and irregular self-monitoring of blood glucose levels (PDRHealth, 2004).

As diabetic adults age, their risk of hypoglycemia increases. They often develop impaired kidney function, and thus are more likely to have altered pharmacokinetics and/or impaired renal glucose production, which will make them vulnerable to prolonged life-threatening hypoglycemia (Chelliah and Burge, 2004; Holstein and Egberts, 2003; Hasslacher and Wittmann, 2003).

Diabetic patients on five or more prescription medications are susceptible to drug-related hypoglycemia. Sulfonylurea, ACE inhibitors and non-selective beta-adrenoceptor antagonists and impaired liver function, all increase the risk for hypoglycemia (Holstein and Egberts, 2003). In addition, hospitalized diabetics with co-morbidities and older diabetics in nursing homes are also vulnerable to hypoglycemic episodes.

Cognitive impairment, a condition which is prevalent in elderly diabetics, can contribute to their lack of understanding of their condition (Raji, et al., 2005; Crooks, et al., 2003). In addition, depression, which is also prevalent in this population can account for a lack of motivation in learning how to avoid hypoglycemic episodes (Bell, et al., 2005).

Based on an 4-year follow-up evaluation of 94 type 1 diabetic patients who participated in a structured 5-day treatment and teaching program, Schiel, et al. (1998) discovered that patients with little knowledge about diabetes had an increased higher HbA1c levels and higher incidence of severe hypoglycemia.

Cardiovascular Risk Factors and Complications

Silent ischemia is prevalent in diabetics, and therefore DM is now frequently viewed as a CHD risk equivalent (Kloner, 2004). Insulin resistance occurs in most glucose disorders in adults and this in turn, increases the risk of cardiovascular disease (Barzilay, et al., 2004b). Persons may have an adverse cardiovascular risk factor profile as a lead-up to non-insulin dependent DM and impaired glucose tolerance (McPhillips, et al., 1990). One investigation of 1,847 men and women, aged 40 to 49 years, who had no known DM or fasting hyperglycemia at the study's baseline, showed that an unfavorable cardiovascular risk factor profile preceded the development of non-insulin dependent DM and impaired glucose tolerance in women and to a lesser extent in men (McPhillips, et al., 1990).

One report from the Cross-Cultural Research on Nutrition in the Older Adult Study Group assessed the prevalence of DM and related coronary risk factors in Mexican populations (Lerman, et al., 1998). They found that diabetes in older Mexicans was related to hypertriglyceridemia and increased rate of ischemic heart disease. Ottenbacher, et al. (2004), drawing on the results of the EPESE, also reported that DM was related to an increased incidence of stroke and mortality in aged Mexican-Americans. In addition, Otiniano, et al. (2002) noted that among elder Mexican-Americans, having had a stroke or a heart attack predicted increased DM-related complications. Lerman, et al. (1998) found that reduced carbohydrate intake, central adiposity, and functional impairment were independent predictors of diabetes mellitus in older Mexicans.

Using a cohort of 829 diabetics, aged 65 and older, in the Cardiovascular Health Study, Barzilay, et al. (2004a) discovered that increased fasting glucose levels predict incident congestive heart failure (CHF). However, they found that the relationship between fasting glucose and CHF is influenced by the presence of coronary heart disease. The association between fasting glucose and CHF was stronger among aged diabetics who did not have CHD at the beginning of the study compared to elder diabetics with baseline CHD. More research is needed to determine if high fasting glucose levels are a risk factor for CHF in adults.

Eye Disease

Aged persons with DM are at high risk of developing vision impairment and eye disease (Brown, et al., 2005; Otiniano, et al., 2002; Sinclair, et al., 2000; Black, et al., 1999). Non-proliferative diabetic retinopathy is one of the most prevalent types of retinopathy seen in patients aged 50 years and older.

Sinclair, et al. (2000) conducted a community-based, case-control study to assess visual impairment in older adults living at home. The study consisted of a population of 386 persons with DM and 385 controls who were age- and sex-matched. The researchers showed that in the general population, age and female sex predicted a greater risk of visual impairment; those with DM had an even greater risk. In addition, in older adults, a history of foot ulcers, a longer duration of DM, and use of insulin were risk factors related to visual impairment.

Eye disease may be particularly common in certain ethnic/cultural and racial groups. For example, Otiniano, et al. (2002), in their study of Mexican-American elders, showed that 38% of the sample reported DM-related eye problems. Diabetic retinopathy has been found to be prevalent in Southern Indian populations. One cross-sectional study of self-reported diabetics, aged 50 and older, in a population of southern India showed that 26.2% of the individuals had diabetic retinopathy (Narendran, et al., 2002). The most prevalent type of diabetic retinopathy found in this sample was non-proliferative diabetic retinopathy.

Kidney Problems

Aged diabetics are particularly vulnerable to nephropathy, also known as diabetic kidney disease. This kidney impairment is due to age-associated deterioration in glomerular filtration and renal damage from DM, hypertension, and other chronic conditions (Hansberry, et al., 2005).

In addition, diabetics are more likely to have nerve damage that impairs their ability to empty the bladder completely, thus giving bacteria the opportunity to cause an infection in the urinary system which can eventually lead to severe kidney problems (PDRHealth, 2004).

Individuals from certain ethnic and racial groups are particularly at risk for developing diabetic kidney disease. African-Americans are 4 times more likely than other groups to develop end-stage renal disease (Albert Einstein Healthcare Network, 2006). In addition, Chasens, et al. (2000) revealed that older African-American diabetics had a higher prevalence of nocturia than those without the disease.

Drawing on data from EPESE, Otiniano, et al. (2002) discovered that 14% of the aged Mexican-Americans in their sample reported having DM-associated kidney problems. Another study of 849 Mexican-Americans, ages 45 and older, in south Texas, found that the diabetics were more likely to suffer kidney or urinary problems than non-diabetics (Bastida, et al., 2001).

Older adults with DM can develop gross proteinuria, which is the presence of abnormally large amounts of protein, usually albumin, in the urine. Persistent proteinuria is usually an indicator of kidney disease. Microalbuminuria and gross proteinuria have been shown to be associated with an increased risk of all-cause mortality in type 2 diabetics. However, little is known about their relationship to cardiovascular mortality. One prospective cohort study by Valmadrid, et al. (2000) evaluated whether microalbuminuria and gross proteinuria are independent predictors of cardiovascular mortality. Using a sample of 840 persons with older-onset DM, the researchers found that 54.8% had normal albuminuria, 24.8% had microalbuminuria, and 20.5% had gross proteinuria. Based on a 1-year follow-up, the investigators discovered that the presence of microalbuminuria, and gross proteinuria predicted both all-cause mortality and mortality from cardiovascular disease, cerebrovascular disease, and CHD. These findings remained after controlling for known cardiovascular risk factors and DM-associated variables.

Marin, et al. (2002) analyzed data from 3,583 patients with type 2 DM and discovered that a serum creatinine of greater or equal to 1.2 mg/dl was found in 15.5% of the patients, and 23.5% of the patients had proteinuria. Diabetic patients with a serum creatinine of greater or equal to 1.2 mg/dl had higher levels of blood pressure and a higher prevalence of cardiovascular disease than those with a serum creatinine level less than 1.2 mg/dl. Diabetic patients with proteinuria had a higher prevalence of cardiovascular disease compared to those without proteinuria.

As noted earlier, older diabetics who are taking medications and who have impaired kidney function are at increased risk of prolonged, potentially fatal hypoglycemia because impaired kidney function disrupts drug elimination (Chelliah and Burge, 2004). Reduction of renal function in patients with type 1 or 2 DM can also produce hypoglycemia due to impaired renal glucose production (Hasslacher and Wittmann, 2003).

According to the United States Renal Data System, diabetics are the fastest growing sub-population of patients with end-stage renal disease (ESRD), and the number of ESRD patients over 60 years old has increased over time (Friedlander and Hricik, 1997). Patients over the age of 65 years are now the fasting growing part of the treated ESRD patient population (Stack and Messana, 2000). Along with this increase, the percentage of ESRD patients with one or more co-morbid health problems has increased from 66% to 85% among diabetic patients and from 57% to 66% among non-diabetic patients. The mortality for patients with ESRD due to DM has decreased in recent decades, although DM is the most prevalent primary condition related to mortality in this patient population.

With the increased growth in the ESRD patient population, it is not surprising that an increased number of patients have begun dialysis or underwent a transplant (Krishnan, et al., 2002). Many of these patients are elderly persons who suffer from co-morbid health problems. Krishnan, et al. (2002) noted that registries worldwide have shown a rapid and strong increase in the percentage of older individuals accepted for renal replacement therapy. Moreover, the number of patients who grow old on dialysis is increasing and this has led to major alterations in the demography of the population of kidney disease patients.

One investigation of 5-year survival of patients with diabetic nephropathy on continuous ambulatory peritoneal dialysis showed that cardiovascular complications increased among both type 1 and type 2 diabetics (Olszowska, et al., 2001). However, type 2 diabetics had a higher ratio of death despite adequate dialysis.

A retrospective, longitudinal cohort study of 12,570 older patients with DM also revealed that mortality rates increased significantly with the progression of chronic kidney disease (Patel, et al., 2005).

Lower Extremity Disease (LED)

Lower extremity disease (LED), such as peripheral arterial disease (PAD) and peripheral insensate neuropathy, is a chronic disease that disproportionately afflicts aged individuals and those with DM (Centers for Disease Control and Prevention (2005a); Kennedy, et al., 2005). A study by the Centers for Disease Control and Prevention (2005a), using the National Health and Nutrition Examination Survey (NHANES), reported that about 18% of individuals, 40 years and older, suffered from LED. The results showed that LED was two times as prevalent among diabetics as among non-diabetics. The study also discovered that about 2/3rd of the individuals with LED and half of the persons with both DM and LED had no symptoms. Persons with LED are at risk of developing life-threatening ulcers, infections gangrene or amputations.

PAD is a chronic, disabling condition and is associated with an increased risk of cardiovascular disease and cerebrovascular ischemic complications (Marso and Hiatt, 2006). When compared to non-diabetics, persons with DM who have PAD have increased risks of suffering ischemic events, all-cause mortality, cardiovascular disease-related mortality and mortality associated with coronary artery disease (Aronow, 2006).

What are the risk factors for PAD and other lower extremity complications among persons with DM? PAD may be related to intermittent claudication or may be associated with critical limb ischemia (Aronow, 2006). People with PAD also may have co-existing coronary artery disease and additional atherosclerotic vascular diseases. Eason, et al. (2005) also found that individuals with DM and a history of smoking at least 1 pack of cigarettes per day have an increased probability of developing asymptomatic PAD.

Researchers are investigating the risk factors for a variety of DM-related lower extremity complications. Based on a study of 3,564 type 2 diabetic patients, De Berardis, et al. (2005) found that insulin treatment, cigarette smoking, low educational level, and the presence of other diabetic complications predicted foot complications.

Circulation problems may be especially prevalent among certain ethnic and racial groups. Based on data from the EPESE, Otiniano, et al. (2002) found that circulation difficulties were the most frequent diabetic complication among 3,050 Mexican-Americans, aged 65 and older. The investigators discovered that 280 or 40% of the Mexican-American elders in the sample reported circulation problems. In addition, they found that 8% of the Mexican-American elders sampled reported having at least one lower extremity amputations. In their study, losing a leg was the most prevalent form of amputation, with 53% of the amputees reporting this type of amputation. During the study follow-up period, 12% of the amputees reported a new amputation and 40% reported had a second amputation during the study follow-up period. The investigators found that 46% of the amputees died during a 5-year follow-up. Otiniano, et al. (2003) also identified factors associated with lower extremity amputation at the start of their study and at a 5-year follow-up. At the beginning of the study, being male, having eye difficulties, having a hip fracture, and having DM for 10 years or more predicted lower extremity amputations. At the five year follow-up it was obesity, having experiencing a stroke, and having DM for 10 years or more that predicted new amputations. Being male and having a history of diabetes were the only common risk factors that predicted lower extremity amputations at both the baseline and 5-year follow-up period.

The incidence of non-traumatic lower extremity amputations is high in hemodialysis patients. Sanchez Perales, et al. (2005) found the incidence of lower extremity amputations to be very high and DM, prior myocardial infarction, and stroke and/or transient ischemic attacks were independent predictors of lower extremity amputations.

Erectile Dysfunction

Studies have revealed that erectile dysfunction is prevalent in elder diabetics. One investigation reported that 75% of men, aged 60 and older, with DM had erectile dysfunction (Kloner, 2004).

It is thought that endothelial dysfunction, advanced atherosclerosis, and diabetic neuropathy are risk factors for erectile dysfunction in persons with DM.

Urinary Incontinence

Aged diabetics may be more likely to suffer urinary incontinence than their non-diabetic peers (California Healthcare Foundation/American Geriatrics Society Panel on Improving Care of Elders with Diabetes, 2003; Brown, et al, 1996; Ueda, et al., 2000).

Diabetics are more likely to experience increased thirst, which can result in drinking more fluids, and thus produce more urinary output. Diabetics can suffer from nerve damage that prevents the bladder from emptying completely, and they may also be unable to sense a full bladder and thus suffer urinary incontinence. They may have stress incontinence in which their bladder leaks after laughing, coughing, or sneezing, or they may develop urge incontinence, which occurs when they have a sudden need to empty the bladder (American Geriatrics Society Foundation for Health in Aging, 2006).

Injurious Falls

After the age of 60, the risks of falling and the severity of injuries from falling increase, resulting in a higher prevalence of morbidity, mortality, and disability (Newton, et al., 2006; California Healthcare Foundation/American Geriatrics Society Panel on Improving Care of Elders with Diabetes, 2003; Tinetti, et al., 1986; Robbins, et al., 1989).

Increased Risk of Joint and Bone Problems and Fractures

Researchers are analyzing the prevalence of joint and bone problems in older diabetics. Based on a stratified random sample of 849 Mexican-American women and men, aged 45 and older, Bastida, et al. (2001) compared 193 diabetics with 656 non-diabetics with regard to medical problems. The investigators discovered that joint and bone problems were more prevalent among Mexican-American diabetics than Mexican-American non-diabetics. Older persons with DM are at increased fracture risk due to more frequent falls, functional impairments, loss of bone mineral density and diabetic complications (Schwartz, et al., 2005; Ottenbacher, et al., 2002).

Pain

Aged persons with DM have a higher probability of developing neuropathic pain than older persons without DM, and older diabetics with pain often go untreated (California Healthcare Foundation/American Geriatrics Society Panel on Improving Care of Elders with Diabetes, 2003; Greene, et al., 1999; Vinik, 1999). One analysis of nursing home residents with DM at the time of admission showed that more that 50% of the nursing home residents with DM were in pain at the time of their admission to the nursing home (Travis, et al., 2004).

Acute Metabolic Emergencies

Elder diabetics are especially vulnerable to certain acute metabolic emergencies, such as hyperglycemia and dehydration, which are the main elements of hyperosmolar hyperglycemic syndrome (Murase, et al., 2006; Gaglia, et al., 2004). Older diabetics are susceptible to this syndrome because with increasing age, insulin secretory reserve, insulin sensitivity, and thirst mechanisms decrease.

When older diabetics develop common illnesses such as a cold or flu, they are at increased risk for hyperglycemia, because of a limited oral intake that can make it more difficult to regulate blood sugars (Murase, et al., 2006). In the geriatric population, the symptoms related to hyperglycemia or hypoglycemia may be difficult to detect. Moreover, these acute complications often occur among individuals who have other chronic DM-related complications thus exacerbating the management of this complicated syndrome.

In addition, aged persons with DM are susceptible to ketoacidosis, another acute complication of DM (Greene, 1986). Elders who suffer from chronic diabetic complications complicate the management of ketoacidosis and increase their risk for morbidity and mortality.

To help avoid these diabetic emergencies, older diabetics should take extra precautions, e.g., maintain their oral intake and monitor blood glucose during common illnesses to avoid these life-threatening crises and receive immediate treatment when symptoms develop (Gaglia, et al., 2004).

Decline in Cognitive Function

Several investigations have shown that cognitive performance in older adults is adversely affected by DM status (Raji, et al., 2005; Kanaya, et al., 2004; Crooks, et al., 2003). One study of 100 consecutive Hispanic-Americans, African-American, and Whites, aged 55 years or older, attending an eye clinic showed that having DM predicted increased cognitive impairment, as measured by the St. Louis Mental Status Examination (SLUMD) scale (Raji, et al., 2005).

Kanaya, et al. (2004) evaluated change in cognitive performance over a four-year period using a sample of 999 white women and men, aged 42 to 89 years, who were part of the Rancho Bernardo Study. In this prospective study, the Mini-Mental State Examination, Verbal Fluency, and Trail-Making Test were employed to measure cognitive performance. Research participants were classified as having normal glucose tolerance, impaired glucose tolerance, or DM. Possible confounding variables, such as total cholesterol, blood pressure, glycohemoglobin level, were evaluated to determine their effects on the relationship between glucose tolerance status and cognitive performance.

The results of this investigation showed that after four years, older white women with DM were four times more likely to suffer major cognitive deterioration in verbal fluency compared to women with normal glucose tolerance or impaired glucose tolerance (Kanaya, et al., 2004). Glycohemoglobin level weakened these results. However, lipid levels, blood pressure, and microvascular or macrovascular disease did not attenuate this effect. The investigators suggest that more effective glucose control might correct this decline in cognitive performance.

Tun, et al. (1987) compared memory self-assessment and performance in older diabetics and non-diabetics to determine whether older persons with DM have more memory problems in their daily activities and if memory self-assessments are associated with cognitive tests performed in the laboratory. Based on a sample of individuals, 55 to 64 years and 65 to 74 years, they found that both DM and increased age predicted worse performance on some cognitive tests as well as increased frequency of self-reported memory problems.

Sinclair, et al. (2000) also evaluated cognitive dysfunction in older diabetics. Based on a case-control study involving 396 older diabetics and 393 non-diabetic matched controls from the All Wales Research into Elderly Study, the researchers found that older persons with type 2 DM demonstrated worse cognitive functioning than older non-diabetics.

DM and Alzheimer's Disease (AD)

The prevalence of Alzheimer's disease (AD) is increasing in older adults, and research indicates that type 2 DM increases the risk of both vascular dementia and AD (Luchsinger, et al., 2005; den Heijer, et al., 2003; Biessels, et al., 2006). Based on a follow-up study of 1,138 individuals with a mean age of 76.2 years, without dementia at the onset of the original study, Luchsinger, et al. (2005) reported that DM, hypertension, heart disease, and current smoking were risk factors for AD. DM and current smoking were the strongest predictors of AD in isolation or in combination with each other.

Researchers are seeking to determine if diabetic vasculopathy increases AD or if DM directly affects AD neuropathology. Based on a population study of older persons, aged 60 to 90 years without dementia, den Heijer, et al. (2003) found that type 2 DM is directly related to hippocampal and amygdalar atrophy, regardless of vascular atrophy. Another study also suggests that non-vascular mechanisms that cause increased atrophy are responsible for the increased risk of AD in persons with type 2 DM.

Depression

Depression is a well-established complication among diabetics (Bell, et al., 2005). Diabetics are twice as likely to develop major depression as non-diabetics (Williams, et al., 2004; Anderson, et al., 2001;

Carney, et al., 1998). Non-insulin dependent DM in older adults is related to an increased rate of depression, and this increased rate of depression is higher than that found in the normal aging population (Tun, et al., 1987).

Depression is linked to greater morbidity, impaired quality of life, and increased rates of mortality among diabetics (Bell, et al., 2005). Black (1999) found that concomitant depressive symptoms in older Mexican-American diabetics were related to higher rates of co-morbid myocardial infarction, hypertension, arthritis, and angina. Moreover, having concomitant symptoms of depression predicted higher rates of diabetic complications, incontinence, vision impairment, and lower perceived health.

Research is underway to assess the prevalence and correlates of depressive symptoms in older adults with DM. Black (1999), using the findings from the EPESE, discovered that 31.1% of the older Mexican-American diabetics reported high rates of symptoms of depression.

Using the results of the Evaluating Long-term Diabetes Self-management among Elder Rural Adults (ELDER) project, Bell, et al. (2005) evaluated the prevalence and predictors of depressive symptoms among 696 rural older African-Americans, Native-Americans, and whites with DM. The investigators discovered that depressive symptoms were associated with gender (female), less than a high school education, being unmarried, increased body mass index, an increased number of chronic health problems, use of multiple prescription medications, and reduced physical functioning. The researchers also found that older diabetics living in rural communities were at risk for depression regardless of their ethnicity or racial background.

Disability and Quality of Life

DM is a risk factor for disability (Wray, et al., 2005; Black, et al., 1999). Diabetics are at greater risk for impaired physical functioning and worse quality of life than older persons without this disease (Caruso, et al., 2000). DM is also a risk factor for lower-extremity disability. Based on a cross-sectional study of 2,873 Mexican-American elderly, Ma, et al. (1998) showed that DM predicted increased impairment in lower-extremity function, e.g., walking across a room and getting from a bed to a chair.

Research is underway to evaluate the possible effects of DM on lower body disability among older Mexican-Americans. One investigation by Al Snih, et al. (2005) assessed the impact of DM and incident lower body disability based on a 7-year follow-up period. They discovered that at the 7-year follow-up, 48.7% of the diabetics who were not disabled at baseline developed impairments in one or more measures of lower extremity functioning. Diabetics were more likely than non-diabetics to have any impairments in lower extremity functioning. Older age and having one or more diabetic complications predicted an increased risk of impairment in mobility and lower extremity-related activities of daily living. The researchers suggest that awareness of lower extremity disability as a potentially modifiable condition and interventions to minimize impairment should be priorities for elder Mexican-American diabetics.

Physical disability has been measured in different ways. One way of classifying physical disability is to combine measures of daily living, mobility, and strength tasks into one composite variable. Wray, et al. (2005) used this classification system and showed that DM was strongly related to subsequent disability in middle-aged and older adults.

Chou and Chi (2005) assessed disability among a random sample of 2,003 older Hong Kong Chinese adults with DM using three measures: 1) basic activities of living (ADLs) (e.g., bathing, dressing, toilet use, and eating), 2) instrumental ADLs (e.g., ability to use telephone, shopping, food preparation, housekeeping, and ability to handle finances, and 3) mobility. The results indicated that older adults with diabetes mellitus had a greater chance of reporting problems in 12 of 15 ADLs than older adults who did not have DM. Older adults with DM were about two times as likely to report problems only in higher functioning tasks or combined problems with both mobility and higher functioning tasks.

Researchers are analyzing which factors best predict higher risk for disability in older persons with DM. 1. Taking insulin: Based on data from the Fremantle Diabetes Study, a prospective, community-based investigation, Bruce, et al. (2005) showed that insulin treatment predicted an increased risk of mobility impairment. 2. Duration of diabetes: Wu, et al., 2003 found that longer duration of DM was related to greater limitation in both basic and instrumental ADLs. 3. Co-morbid conditions: Using a sample of 1,238 persons with type 2 DM who were 55 years of age or older and enrolled in the Type II Diabetes Patient Outcomes Research Team, Caruso, et al. (2000) found that increased co-morbid health problems was one of the risk factors for disability in type 2 diabetics. Some of these co-morbid conditions are: end stage renal disease, depression, cognitive impairment, sleep disturbances, stroke.

Depression can severely impair cognitive functioning in older diabetics. Tun, et al. (1987) showed that depression was a better predictor of self-reported memory problems than the DM variable. Independent of depression or negative affect, positive affect or emotional well-being in older individuals with DM may predict subsequent functional independence and survival. A 2-year prospective cohort study of 2,282 Mexican Americans, aged 65 to 99, found that positive affect predicted lower rates of mobility impairment and mortality (Ostir, et al., 2000).

Based on a sample of 3,050 Mexican-Americans, aged 65 or older, Otiniano, et al. (2003) found that DM in combination with stroke predicted increased risk of disability among the elder Mexican-Americans.

DM-associated lower extremity complications, such as neuropathic pain, ulcers, lower extremity infections, hip fractures, and amputations are also risk factors for disability in older adults with DM.

The Centers for Disease Control and Prevention (2005b) evaluated mobility limitation among individuals, aged 40 years or older with and without DM and LED. On the basis of the National Health and Nutrition Examination Survey, the researchers showed that there was a higher prevalence of mobility limitation among individuals having either DM or LED than among persons without the diseases. Moreover, individuals with both conditions had a higher prevalence of mobility limitation than individuals with either disease alone.

Sinclair, et al. (2000) showed that impaired visual acuity was linked to significant impairments in physical and social functioning, emotional well-being, vitality and perceptions of health.

Socioeconomic factors have been found to be predictive of disability in older adults with DM. For example, in Caruso, et al. (2000)'s study, lower educational level was associated with a higher prevalence of disability in older adults with type 2 DM.

Obesity has been found to be a risk factor for disability in older adults with type 2 DM (Goya Wannamethee, et al., 2004; Caruso, et al., 2000). Using the results of the Type II Patient Outcomes

Research Team project, Caruso, et al. (2000) evaluated the association between obesity and physical functioning. Based on the PFI-10, a 10-item scale of physical function from the Short-Form-36 Health Survey (SF-36), the researchers showed that obesity predicted worse functioning in type 2 diabetics, aged 55 years and older.

Another report assessed the effects of overweight and obesity on disease burden and disability in elderly men drawing on data from 4,232 men, aged 60 to 79 years (Goya Wannamethee, et al., 2004). According to the results, obese elderly men were almost three times as likely to have DM. The researchers reported that over 60% of the patients with major insulin resistance were associated with overweight and obesity, a third of the patients with DM and hypertension, one fourth of the patients with locomotor disability, and a fifth of the patients with major cardiovascular disease.

In Caruso, et al. (2000)'s study, lack of regular exercise was associated with an increase in impaired physical functioning. In addition, data from the Fremantle Diabetes Study were used to evaluate the possible impact of exercise in influencing mobility and physical disability in patients with type 2 DM (Bruce, et al., 2005). The investigators discovered that participating in exercise and being married reduced the risk of mobility impairment.

Caruso, et al. (2000) discovered that abstinence from alcohol was related to higher prevalence of disability in older persons with type 2 DM.

In order to promote better functional status in older persons with type 2 DM, the investigators recommend regular exercise, weight loss, and treatment for depression. In addition, moderate alcohol use may be helpful.

Stress, Coping, and Social Support

Psychosocial Stress

Diabetics of all ages can experience severe psychosocial stress and related anxiety and depression (Bell, et al., 2005; Williams, et al., 2004; Centers for Disease Control and Prevention, 2004; Herpertz, et al., 2000). The Centers for Disease Control and Prevention (CDC) evaluated the prevalence of serious psychological distress among persons with DM in New York City using data from about 10,000 adults from the 2003 New York City Community Health

Survey. The CDC discovered that adults with DM were two times as likely to have serious psychological distress (e.g., depression, anxiety, and other disorders causing serious psychological distress) as non-diabetics. The findings also revealed that those diabetics with serious psychological distress were more likely than persons with only DM to be poor, have low perceived health, have poor access to health care, and to have experienced spouse or partner loss through separation, divorce, or death.

A study in Germany of 157 patients with type 1 DM and 253 patients with type 2 DM revealed that 16.6% of the sample had extreme psychosocial stress scores (Herpertz, et al., 2000). The authors showed that the use of insulin in patients with type 2 DM, but not the type of treatment, had an impact on psychosocial stress. Patients who were under extreme psychosocial stress were more likely to have worse metabolic control compared to those who were under less psychosocial stress. In patients with both type 1 and type 2 DM, extreme psychosocial stress was related to depression. In type 1 diabetics, extreme psychosocial stress was associated with fear of hypoglycemic episodes, while in type 2 diabetics, maximum psychosocial stress was related to physical health problems.

Psychosocial stress, itself, influences the development of DM. It can impair glycemic control and be a cause or consequence of diabetic complications. Psychosocial stress also can worsen existing DM by limiting the person's capacity to manage their disease (Schoenberg, et al., 2005).

Various protocols have been designed to analyze psychosocial adaptation and the effects of psychosocial stress on diabetics. These instruments include the Problem Areas in Diabetes (PAID) protocol, the Questionnaire on Stress in Patients with Diabetes (revised) (QSD-R) and the Diabetes Quality of Life Scale have been used (Gabbay, et al., 2006; Herpertz, et al., 2000; Trief, et al., 1998).

Using the PAID, West and McDowell (2003) evaluated sources of distress experienced by persons with DM. They discovered that sources of distress included worrying about the future, worrying about the potential for diabetic complications, and feeling guilty about being non-compliant with their diabetic regimen. Other factors that impacted distress consisted of the type of treatment, duration of DM, and age.

Older individuals with DM are especially vulnerable to various stressors. They can suffer from stress related to the burden of daily life, the difficulties in complying with nutritional therapy, and problems in following drug treatment. The Elderly Diabetes Impact Scale has been constructed to evaluate the stressful consequence of the disease on aged individuals (Araki, et al., 1995).

As a consequence of these multiple stressors, aged persons with DM can experience a worsening of diabetic complications which, in turn can cause severe psychosocial distress. Moreover, aged diabetics are at increased risk of suffering from number of stress-related illnesses such as sleep disturbances, gastrointestinal problems, and back problems (Chasens, et al., 2000; Han, et al., 2002). Psychosocial stress has also been linked to lower perceived health and quality of life.

Coping

Individuals may use a variety of strategies in coping with DM and other chronic illnesses. They may cope with their condition by seeking information about their condition, by expressing emotions, and/or by minimizing the threat of the condition.

In an attempt to determine if age makes a difference when coping with chronic disease, Felton and Revenson (1987) evaluated whether there age differences in coping with chronic diseases used a sample of 151 middle-aged and older adults with chronic illnesses. They examined six coping techniques: cognitive restructuring, expressing emotions, wish fulfilling fantasy, self-blame, seeking information, and minimizing threats. The results indicated that age affects the ways in which people adapt to chronic conditions. Older adults were less likely than younger people to express emotions or seek information. Older individuals who felt that their disease was very serious tended to minimize the threat, avoid researching their disease, and have wish-fulfilling fantasies about their situation.

Family and Social Support

Family and social support can help aged diabetics follow their diet, exercise, blood glucose monitoring, and foot self-care practices by motivating them, offering instruction, and obtaining necessary equipment and other resources (Wen, et al., 2004).

Penninx, et al. (1998) evaluated the effects of social support and personal coping resources on depression in older adults with DM and other chronic diseases. The authors discovered that having a partner, have many close relationships, greater self-mastery, expectations for self-efficacy, and high self-esteem predicted less depressive symptoms. In elder diabetics, having received instrumental support, e.g., receiving information about their disease was related to having more depressive symptoms.

Wen, et al. (2004) used a sample of 138 adults, aged 55 years and older to analyze the impact of family support on exercise and diet among older Mexican-Americans with type 2 DM. They discovered that individuals with higher levels of self-reported family support were more likely to follow their diet and exercise program. Older diabetics who reported more barriers to exercise were less likely to engage in exercise.

Samuel-Hodge, et al. (2005) surveyed 299 older African-American women with type 2 DM and found that the greater the number of adults living in the household, the greater the barrier to adequate self care, because of the women's inability to say "no". In contrast, Wen, et al. (2004) discovered that among older Mexican-Americans with type 2 DM, living with a larger number of family members was related to an increased chance of adhering to a diet and exercise program. Ethnic/racial and cultural differences in family dynamics may help to account for these inconsistencies.

Based on a national sample of African-American, Hispanic and white diabetics and non-diabetics, 60 years and older, Bertera (2003) reported that Mexican-Americans and other Hispanics reported the lowest levels of social support and affiliation on four out of five measures.

In addition to problems in the quality of family and social support, the total absence of that support interferes with the ability of elder diabetics to adhere to their medical regimen. Older diabetics who live alone after many years of living with a spouse or companion may have problems living alone, particularly at mealtimes (U.S. Food and Drug Administration, 1996). These people may suffer depression and lose interest in preparing regular meals or eating or they may eat only small amounts of food on an irregular basis. This is particularly problematic since elder diabetics frequently need to prepare and eat special diets.

A study of newly widowed people, most of whom were women, showed that they were less likely to report enjoying their meals, less likely to have a good appetite, and less likely to have good eating habits, compared to married persons (U.S. Food and Drug Administration, 1996). Widowed persons tended to lose an average of 7.6 pounds during the two years after a spouse's death.

Most of the women in the study, reported having enjoyed cooking and eating when they were married. However, since they have been widowed, they have viewed cooking and eating as chores, particularly since there is no one to enjoy their cooking (U.S. Food and Drug Administration, 1996).

Many widowed men who were unaccustomed to cooking may not know how to prepare meals and therefore be more likely to eat out or have snacks. This regime may result in eating high fat- and high-cholesterol food, which do not contain an adequate amount of vitamins and minerals (U.S. Food and Drug Administration, 1996).

Treatment and Rehabilitation Outcomes

The following risk factors should be examined when making treatment decisions for older diabetics: age; life expectancy; co-morbid health problems; and psychosocial problems, such as anxiety and depression, for they all have an impact on the older diabetic patients' ability to follow dietary, exercise, medication, and stress management regimens (Rosenstock, 2001).

The goal of treatment should be to improve the patient's clinical status and quality of life (Smitz, 2005; Rosenstock, 2001). Treatment of older adults with DM should emphasize education (See Patient Education and Self-Management in this chapter), glycemic control, modifying cardiovascular risk factors, eye care, foot care, and managing nephropathy and geriatric syndromes. A team approach is the best way to provide comprehensive treatment for these at-risk individuals.

Glycemic Control

Achieving glycemic control and reducing cardiovascular risk factors can reduce the complications of DM in older adults and enhance their quality of life (Chelliah and Burge, 2004; Smitz, 2005; Rosenstock, 2001).

Treatment objectives are aimed at achieving glycemic control in a structured approach that consists of non-pharmacological technique and pharmacological therapy (Rosenstock, 2001). Non-pharmacological methods include diet, exercise, and psychosocial stress management, while pharmacological therapy includes oral anti-hyperglycemic agents by themselves or in combination with insulin.

Diet for Aged Diabetics

A nutritional plan for aged diabetics should involve one or more of the following recommendations. First, individuals should lose weight if they are overweight (White, 2002). Losing 5 to 10 pounds can enhance metabolic control in individuals who are overweight. These persons frequently have type 2 DM.

Second, aged diabetics should lower their saturated fat and cholesterol to achieve better cardiovascular health (White, 2002). These individuals can reduce their caloric intake by lowering their total fat intake and thus help them control their weight and manage type 2 DM and other conditions that increase their risks for developing coronary heart disease. The third Report of the National Cholesterol Education Program recommends that total fat intake should be less than 30% and saturated fat (e.g., solid vegetable shortening, milk fat in whole milk and cheeses, poultry skin, and animal fats) should be less than 10% of total daily calories, and cholesterol intake should be limited to less than 300mg/d. All diabetics should be encouraged to follow these guidelines.

In his study of 10,066 women, aged 45 years and older, Liu, et al. (2005) discovered that intakes of calcium and dairy products predicted a lower prevalence of the metabolic syndrome (obesity associated health risks for diabetes, coronary artery disease and stroke) in women who were middle age and older.

Third, older persons if hypertensive should reduce their sodium intake to less than 2.3 g of sodium (or about 1 tsp of salt) per day (White, 2002). Individuals with hypertension, especially in those who are aged or African-American, who reduce their sodium intake to this level can help attenuate the rise systolic blood pressure related to age, reduce systolic blood pressure and diastolic blood pressure in many persons with hypertension, and reduce or eliminate the need for medication.

Fourth, aged diabetics should increase their intake of dietary fiber from a variety of foods to 20 to 35 g per day (White, 2002).

Fifth, diabetics should follow a meal plan that is based on a regular pattern of food intake and preferences (White, 2002). The amount of carbohydrate, protein and fat content in their meal plan should be determined based on their health problems and treatment goals. This customized meal plan is especially important for older individuals with type 1 DM.

Sixth, these individuals should eliminate or limit their intake of alcohol to 24 oz. of beer, 8 oz. of wine or 2 oz. of 100- proof distilled spirits (White, 2002). For women, the U.S. Dietary Guidelines for Americans recommends that their intake of alcohol should be less than half of that listed in this recommendation.

Finally, it is recommended that aged diabetics stop smoking (White, 2002).

The above nutritional recommendations also should be implemented for persons who have impaired glucose tolerance or impaired fasting glucose even if they do not have frank DM (White, 2002). In addition, these recommendations may be appropriate for individuals from minority groups who have a greater risk of developing type 2 DM than whites.

Exercise and Older Diabetics

Bell (1992) notes that an exercise program can help both type 1 and type 2 diabetics improve lipid assessments, reduce blood pressure and weight, and enhance other cardiovascular risk factors. Pescatello, et al. (2000) used a cross-sectional observational study of 155 healthy, older adults living at home to evaluate the effects of low-intensity physical activity on blood lipids and lipoproteins. The findings revealed that low-intensity physical activity is related to improved blood lipids and lipoproteins in older adults. Smitz (2005) found that exercise is also associated with reduced mortality from all causes and cardiovascular mortality.

Aged diabetics should participate in age-and abilities-appropriate physical activity (Jack, et al., 2004). Those diabetics capable of engaging in exercise should participate in both resistance exercise and aerobic exercise. These two forms of exercise help to maintain metabolic control and prevent depression, atherosclerosis, osteoporosis, and other disorders (Araki, 2006; Ryan,

2001). Exercise can also help diabetics prevent other diabetic complications (Oshida and Ishiguro, 2006). However, there are risks associated with exercise for older diabetics. They may suffer an adverse cardiovascular event, damage to the soft tissue and joints of the feet, visual loss, early and delayed hypoglycemia, and hyperglycemia and ketosis. Before prescribing an exercise program, clinicians should perform a comprehensive evaluation, identifying possible diabetic complications and determine the patient's level of fitness. Careful attention to insulin doses and glucose monitoring can help avoid problems with glycemic control. (Bell, 1992)

After thorough medical evaluations, aged diabetics should begin with mild aerobic exercise, such as walking, cycling, and swimming to improve their insulin-signaling pathway (Oshida and Ishiguro, 2006). Aerobic exercise must be performed at least three days a week and should last 20 to 45 minutes (White, 2002). The patients should include low-intensity warm-up and cool-down exercises. If aerobic exercise by itself is ineffective, then the next step in an aerobic regime would be engaging in resistance exercise (Oshida and Ishiguro, 2006). This type of exercise, which includes rowing and lifting weights, increases skeletal muscle volume and strength. The combination of aerobic and resistance exercises improves both insulin resistance and quality of life for older individuals with DM (Oshida and Ishiguro, 2006; Bell, 1992).

The use of appropriate footwear and other protective equipment is essential (White, 2002). Diabetics should inspect their feet daily after exercise, and they should avoid exercise if they are experiencing poor glycemic control.

Psychosocial Stress Management of Aged Diabetics

As described earlier, older diabetics are vulnerable to stress, especially DM-related stress, and are at increased risk for depression and other psychosocial problems, and, therefore, psychosocial stress management is vital for these individuals.

The Centers for Disease Control and Prevention recommend an integrated program of health care, both physical and mental health care services, to respond to serious psychosocial stress in persons with DM (Centers for Disease Control and Prevention, 2004).

Jack, et al. (2004) recommend a partnership between aged diabetics and clinicians. This collaborative care management approach assumes that patients are experts about their lives and health care provider are experts about the disease process. They note that this type of partnership can help health professionals treat severe psychosocial distress and cognitive impairment in this group.

Williams, et al. (2004) evaluated the effectiveness of a depression care management program on DM-associated outcomes in patients, 60 years of age or older. The intervention consisted of a care manager who provided education, problem-solving therapy, and/or support for antidepressant management using a primary care physician. The program evaluation showed that the participants suffered less severe depression and better improvement in functioning than did those who received standard care. Patients in the intervention group had an increase in the number of days exercised weekly, but other self-care activities and glycemic control did not change.

Katon, et al. (2006) assessed the cost-effectiveness and net benefit of this program and found that the intervention produced a net benefit of $1,129. The investigators concluded that the depression care management program offered significant clinical benefits at a cost that is no greater than standard care for older diabetics.

Based on a randomized-controlled trial, Gabbay, et al. (2006) analyzed the impact of one nurse case management program on diabetics' emotional distress and other outcomes. The program included self-management education and the initiation of DM guidelines. The authors found that after participating in the intervention group, the diabetics were more likely to have reduced blood pressure and lower DM-associated emotional distress than diabetics in the control group.

Drug Therapy

When selecting an appropriate pharmacological therapy, clinicians should take into account age-associated changes in pharmacokinetics and the potential for adverse drug effects and interactions (Rosenstock, 2001). A conservative and step-by-step approach is recommended for pharmacological therapy for older adults with type

2 DM. Treatment may be started with monotherapy. This can be followed by a combination of oral agents, including sulphonylurea as a foundation insulin secretagogue in addition to a supplemental insulin sensitizer. If significant hyperglycemia (glycosylated hemoglobin or HbA1c is greater than 8%) persists despite oral combination therapy, insulin therapy is eventually necessary. Therefore, clinicians should make sure that their goals for glycemic control and HbA1c are realistic, flexible, and customized to the characteristics of the older adult diabetic patients.

The use of anti-hyperglycemic agents and other drugs can produce severe or fatal hypoglycemia and the risk of drug-related hypoglycemia increases with age and co-morbid health problems (Rosenstock, 2001). It is important to identify all of the causes of the hypoglycemia and then design and initiate a prevention plan (Chelliah and Burge, 2004). A global evaluation of the patient should be undertaken to identify possible risk factors. Once risk factors have been identified, target glycemic goals should be customized to the unique characteristics of the older patient. Clinicians should carefully select anti-diabetic agents based their assessment of the patient's unique characteristics and risk factors. Patients and their families should be educated to recognize and treat hypoglycemic episodes. Finally, care should be coordinated between clinicians, patients and families to identify, treat, and prevent hypoglycemia.

Treatment of Cardiovascular Disease in Older Adults with DM

Reducing cardiovascular risk factors is essential since cardiovascular complications are the primary cause of morbidity and mortality in older persons with DM (Smitz, 2005). It is important to treat hypertension gradually. The treatment regimen for this population consists of changing the patients' lifestyle, prescribing anti-hyperglycemic medications and routine evaluations to assess and review their current medications.

Unfortunately, older adult may not receive optimal treatment for their cardiovascular risk factors. One investigation by Smith, et al. (2002) assessed cardiovascular risk-factor treatment and control using data from a population-based, prospective cohort of older people with and without DM. The authors discovered that management of cardiovascular risk factors was deficient, especially among persons with DM. Among individuals with hypertension, diabetics were more likely than non-diabetics to be treated with anti-hypertensive medications (89% vs. 75%). However, diabetics were less likely than non-diabetics to have recommended blood pressure levels of 139/89 mmHg or lower (27% vs. 48%). Diabetic dyslipidemic persons were less likely to be treated with lipid-lowering medication (26% vs. 55%) and achieved recommended treatment goals less frequently (8% vs. 54%) than non-diabetic dyslipidemic persons.

Eye Care

Routine eye care is essential to minimize the risk and complications of diabetic retinopathy in older adults and this to improve their life expectancy and quality of life (Smitz, 2005). Unfortunately, various studies have shown that eye care for many diabetics is sub-optimal in the U.S (Centers for Disease Control and Prevention, 2005; Hollander, et al., 2005). The quality of eye care seems to be directly related to the funding of health services. Hollander, et al. (2005) studied large fee-for-service primary care group practices and discovered that only 16% of the patients were given eye exams. In contrast, the researchers found that 63% of the Medicare patients had an annual eye examination.

Foot Care

Routine foot care is also necessary to avoid potentially fatal lower extremity amputations, ulcers, and other lower extremity complications. According to Helfand (2003), the first element of preventing foot problems in older diabetics is patient education. Clinicians should fully inform the patients and their caretakers of the nature of foot problems and self-management processes. It is critical that the patients be open to changing their lifestyle to prevent lower extremity complications.

   Nicolucci, et al. (1996) illustrated the importance of patient education in his study of 866 patients with long-term DM-related complications and 1,888 controls. They found that patients who did not receive DM education had an increased the likelihood of suffering DM-associated complications.

The second element of prevention is the on-going surveillance and management of foot problems and diabetic complications among high risk diabetics by health care professionals (Helfand, 2003). This process facilitates an early identification of complications and secondary prevention of chronic conditions. Since Medicare now covers footwear and orthotics for at-risk diabetics, the probabilities are high that referrals for podiatric care will be followed.

Unfortunately, deficits in foot diagnosis and care have been found. In 2002 to 2004, a Centers for Disease Control and Prevention study found that only four in 10 diabetic adults reported having had an annual foot examination, an annual dilated eye examination, and a hemoglobin A1c test. Hollander, et al., (2005), in his investigation of 2,010 Medicare patients with DM revealed that only 49% of the patients had received an annual foot examination.

De Berardis, et al. (2005) also found problems in the delivery of foot care to type 2 diabetic patients in 2005. Their study revealed that 50% of the patients reported that their physician had not examined their feet in the last year. Moreover, it was the general practitioners who were less likely to conduct foot examinations on these high risk patients who had diabetic neuropathy or peripheral vascular disease.

Some health care professionals seem to be unaware that their diabetic patients are at risk for developing life-threatening lower extremity complications when they present with peripheral neuropathy, peripheral vascular disease, or a prior foot ulcer. Based on a case-control study at a Veterans Affair Medical Center, authors found that peripheral neuropathy or peripheral vascular disease was related to a risk of lower extremity amputation. However, patients with either of these two diseases were no more likely to receive medical care or self-care instruction than those who had neither of these two diseases (Del Aguila, et al., 1994).

The investigators did find that patients who had a history of a foot ulcer were more likely to receive medical care or patient education than those without this condition.

Health professional education offers the possibility of improving diabetic care, but the impact of training on diabetic clinical practice and the patient care outcomes remains to be determined. An investigation by Bruckner, et al. (1999) evaluated the impact of Project LEAP, a statewide health professional training program, on the prevention of lower extremity amputations in individuals with type 2 DM. Project LEAP consisted of 27 1-day workshops offered to 560 clinicians from 85 health care organizations. The program evaluation revealed that the clinicians improved their provision of foot-care patient education, documentation of peripheral vascular disease, documentation of patients' preventive self-care practices, and appropriate referrals to podiatrists and other health care professionals. While the overall incidence of lower extremity amputations had no significant change, there were fewer amputations among patients in hospitals and community healthcare organizations than for residents in nursing homes and rehabilitation facilities.

Management of Kidney Problems

Identifying and managing kidney problems are important aspects in the treatment of older adults with DM (Smitz, 2005). The treatment for nephropathy should emphasize slowing the progression of kidney failure. This can be achieved by controlling blood pressure and blood glucose levels, participating in medically-supervised exercise, weight loss, and following a diabetic diet (Albert Einstein Healthcare Network, 2006).

Practice guidelines recommend achieving a blood pressure target of less than 130/80 mmHG to conservatively treat chronic kidney disease. In Italy, De Nicola, et al. (2005) evaluated a sample of 1,201 adult non-dialyzed patients with chronic kidney disease, and found that in 88% of the patients the blood pressure target of less than 130/80 mmHG was not attained.

Another report, based on 12, 570 older patients with DM treated within a Veterans Affairs network revealed that only 32% of patients with an estimated glomerular filtration rate of 15 to 29 mL/min/1.73 m2 had been treated in a nephrology clinic (Patel, et al., 2005). These authors suggest that the under recognition of chronic kidney disease may be due to a reliance on serum creatinine levels in aged diabetic patients, thus overestimating their kidney function.

Older diabetics can benefit from a referral to a nephrology clinic. Lynn, et al. (2005), in a retrospective study of patients, aged 65 or older, referred to a nephrology clinic, found that 50% of the patients changed their disease management strategies after their clinic visit.

Management of Geriatric Syndromes

Older adults with DM are especially susceptible to geriatric syndromes, such as dehydration, cognitive impairment, and depression (Smitz, 2005; Gaglia, et al., 2004). Therefore, it is mandatory to identify and manage these syndromes in order to enhance the patients' life expectancy and quality of life.

Patient Education and Self-Management

DM education for the elderly should be customized to meet the individual needs of this heterogeneous patient population (Matsuoka, 2006). Araki (2006) notes that DM education should emphasize glycemic control and quality of life, because of their co-morbid health problems, related impairments, and additional risk factors for atherosclerosis and cardiovascular disease (Zeyfang, 2005; Matsuoka, 2006). In addition, developing educational programs and treatment plans should take into account the patients' own views about their disease and treatment strategies (Ishii, 2006).

Simple practical nutrition education for this population should concentrate on maintaining nutritional balance instead of emphasizing caloric restriction.

Older diabetics should receive comprehensive foot care education and should inspect their feet on a regular basis. De Berardis, et al. (2005) discovered that 28% of type 2 diabetics in a study had not received foot care education, and 33% reported that they had not examined their feet.

Another part of DM education is to promote both resistance exercise and aerobic exercise, which helps to promote metabolic control and prevent diseases, such as depression, atherosclerosis, osteoporosis, and sarcopenia (Araki, 2006). In addition, DM education should also emphasize blood glucose self-testing as a means of helping the patients deal with and/or prevent hypoglycemia, hyperglycemia, or periods of sickness. Patients should be taught how to follow sliding rules of insulin dose in the event of unstable nutritional intake.

Older persons may be particularly at risk because they may be unaware of elevated serum glucose levels. Bertera (2003), using a national sample of Hispanics, African-Americans, and whites, discovered that Mexican-Americans, along with whites, were more likely to be unaware that their serum glucose level was greater than 115 mg/dl. A survey of Chinese patients with DM revealed that only half of the patients had adequate knowledge about their condition. Factors such as educational level, longer duration of the disease, and presence of diabetic complications have been shown to be related to the patients' knowledge about diabetes (T'ang, et al., 1999).

Aged individuals with DM and related complications may face a number of barriers in participating in and benefiting from DM education programs (Rhee, et al., 2005). Some of these barriers are:

1. Diabetic retinopathy with its accompanying visual impairments and difficulty in reading.
2. Cognitive difficulties, which result in an inability to follow a complex regimen, including diet, medication, self-monitoring of blood sugar, foot care, and exercise (Schiel, et al., 2004; Braun, et al., 2004; Raji, et al., 2005; Kanaya, et al., 2004; Crooks, et al., 2003).
3. Depression which interferes with their knowledge of diabetes and reduces their motivation and energy to follow a complex diabetic regimen (Bell, et al., 2005).
4. Race and ethnicity - Schoenberg and Drungle (2001) found that older African-American women with DM were more likely than older white women to report that finances, pain, and visual impairments were obstacles to performing self-management. However, both older African-American and white women indicated that they were reluctant to self-monitor blood glucose and exercise (Schoenberg and Drungle, 2001).
5. Low socioeconomic status - A study of self-monitoring of blood glucose among adults with DM in an HMO revealed that lower socioeconomic status based on residence, older age, and other factors were associated with lower rates of self-monitoring (Adams, et al., 2003). A pilot study of low income urban Puerto Ricans by von Goeler, et al. (2003) evaluated obstacles to self-management. The individuals surveyed were older, had limited education, but good access to health care. A majority of them indicated that they had limited knowledge about DM, did not follow their diabetic regimen, and had negative attitudes about DM.
6. Educational Level - Rhee, et al. (2005) also assessed the role of educational level as a barrier to attending DM training. The researchers showed that having an elementary education or less was related with lower rates of participating in DM education.

7. Obesity - Adams, et al. (2003) discovered that obesity was related to lower rates of self-monitoring of blood glucose and to a lower likelihood of attending DM education programs (Rhee, et al., 2005).

In addition, to demographic, socioeconomic, and lifestyle factors, Schoenberg, et al. (1998) discovered that older women with type 2 DM who believed that they had developed DM because of their prior diet, because they were currently overweight, or because they had abnormal bodily functioning had a greater likelihood of following their diabetic regimen.

Dye, et al. (2003) used focus groups to analyze factors that influence diet and exercise among persons, over the age of 55, with DM. Their results indicated that willpower, often derived from a belief in God, is essential for positive behavioral change. The authors also found that changing unhealthy behaviors and improving self-efficacy begins with small steps and intrinsic reinforcement is a precondition for behavior modification.

Since diabetic patients, may suffer cognitive impairment and have less capacity for self-management, researchers are evaluating the effectiveness of DM education in helping then deal with cognitive dysfunction. Schiel, et al. (2004) and Braun, et al. (2004) evaluated the effectiveness of a specialized structured treatment and teaching program in Germany, known as Dikol, that emphasizes insulin therapy and takes into account impaired cognitive function among type 2 diabetics. Dikol offers more practical exercises for diabetics and less time on theoretical topics, such as pathophysiology, insulin action, and calculating nutritional needs. Based on a sample of 106 type 2 diabetic patients with the mean age of 68.6 years and median DM duration of 10.3 years, Schiel, et al. (2004) showed that patients in the Dikol program had similar quality of metabolic control and knowledge of DM as the patients in the standard patient education group. However, patients in Dikol program did better in their self-management than those in the standard patient education intervention. In addition, those in the Dikol intervention tended to need less assistance from others than those in the usual patient education program. Dikol patients expressed more satisfaction with their education and therapy than did patients in the usual patient education program. Neither group had acute complications, such as foot ulcers, hypoglycemia, and coma.

As noted previously, families and friends can help elder diabetics cope with the psychosocial effects of their disease and facilitate patient compliance with their regimen (Wen, et al., 2004).

Research has been underway to assess the extent to which DM support groups can enhance the effectiveness of patient education outcomes in aged diabetics. A pilot study by Gilden, et al. (1992) compared patients who attended a patient education program that was followed by 18 months of support group activities with two control groups, one group who attended only a patient education program and the other who did not participate in either intervention. The authors found that those who participated in the educational program followed by support group sessions had better knowledge of DM, reduced stress, increased family participation, and better metabolic control than patients in the other two groups.

The use of facilitated telephone peer support for older adults with DM has been evaluated. Heisler and Piette (2005) examined the feasibility and acceptability of employing an Interactive Voice Response (IVR)-based system to promote peer support among older diabetics. Participants in the intervention were asked to contact their partner weekly using the toll-free IVR calling line. The pilot findings revealed that 73% reported that their partner had helped them enhance their self-care practices, and 70% reported that they had helped their partner engage in appropriate behaviors to maintain health.

Gilden, et al. (1989) showed that a 6-week DM education program for older patients and their spouses increased DM knowledge, reduced stress levels, enhanced diet-related quality of life, increased family involvement, and improved glycemic control, compared to older diabetic patients without participating spouses. The results also indicated that the intervention increased the spouses' DM knowledge and perceived involvement in the care of their diabetic spouses.

7
Rheumatoid Arthritis, Osteoarthritis, Osteoporosis, Fibromyalgia, and Low Back Pain in Older Adults

Complications and Risk Factors

Arthritis

Arthritis is the most prevalent chronic condition and the most frequent cause of disability among older adults in the U.S. (Verbrugge and Juarez, 2006). Many arthritic individuals have co-morbidities, a fact substantiated by Stang, et al.'s (2006) evaluation of the data from the National Co-morbidity Survey Replication. He found that 27.3% of the persons interviewed reported having arthritis. About 81% of these individuals had at least one other physical or mental problem, including 45.6% who had other chronic pain problems, 62.3% with chronic physical conditions, and 24.3% with mental disorders.

Aged adults with arthritis in their feet, legs and/or knees, are at increased risk for falls and related injuries. Based on a sample of 684 men and women, aged 75-89 years, living in the community, Sturnieks, et al. (2004) discovered that elder adults with lower extremity arthritis had a higher probability of falls, including falls, (some associated with injuries). The increased risk of falling was associated with reduced knee extension strength and increased postural sway.

Below is a discussion of complications, co-morbidity, and disease progression associated with different types of arthritis and musculoskeletal disorders.

Rheumatoid Arthritis (RA)

Rheumatoid arthritis (RA) is a diffuse connective tissue disease and is a multi-system disorder with an inflammatory process initially affecting joints. The first signs of the disease usually occur in individuals, aged 35 to 50. RA is a major cause of disability in older adults, who in addition, frequently have a number of chronic co-morbidities. In a study of 186 patients with recent onset of RA, Kroot, et al. (2001) found that 27% of the patients had at least one other chronic condition. The most frequently reported co-morbidities were cardiovascular disease (29%), respiratory disease (18%), or dermatological conditions (11%).

Using several population-based prevalence cohorts of RA patients, Gabriel, et al. (1999) showed that these patients had an increased risk of acquiring congestive heart disease, chronic lung disease, dementia, and peptic ulcer disease. The authors also discovered that age, male gender, and baseline co-morbidity predicted an increased rate of co-morbid health problems.

Persons with RA may suffer neurological pathology, including cervicocranialgia, cervical myelopathy, pathological alterations in the upper cervical spine, and cerebral problems (Klin Med, 2006).

In addition, people with RA may be more susceptible to developing infections. Using a population-based incidence cohort study of 609 RA patients, Doran, et al. (2002) discovered that 64% had suffered at least one recent infection. Increasing age, extraarticular disease manifestations of RA, leucopenia, co-morbidities, and use of corticosteroids were associated with an increased risk of infection.

RA patients are at increased risk for cardiovascular disease and coronary heart disease, including acute myocardial infarction (Roman, et al., 2006; Maradit-Kremers, et al., 2005a; Krishnan, et al., 2004). Maradit-Kremers, et al. (2005b) used longitudinal, population-based data to assess whether systemic inflammation increases the risk of cardiovascular death in RA patients. Their results indicated that a history of coronary heart disease, smoking, hypertension, low body mass index, and diabetes mellitus predicted increased risk of cardiovascular death in these patients. In addition, various RA co-morbidities, including peripheral vascular disease, cerebrovascular disease, chronic pulmonary disease, dementia, ulcers, cancer, renal disorders, liver disease, and history of alcoholism were associated with an increased risk of cardiovascular death.

Older RA individuals may be at increased risk of atherosclerosis as shown in a case-control study by Roman, et al. (2006) which demonstrated that age predicted the development of carotid atherosclerotic plaque in RA patients.

Based on a study of 631 patients with RA, del Rincon, et al. (2005) showed that both cardiovascular risk factors and RA disease indicators predict carotid atherosclerosis. However, cardiovascular risk factors were more likely to occur in the older patients, while clinical indicators of RA disease were more likely to develop in the younger patients.

RA patients have a higher risk of death than that expected in the general population (Gabriel, et al., 2003). Because of its association with cardiovascular disease, RA is related to increased morbidity and mortality (Roman, et al., 2006).

A population-based study of RA patients by Maradit-Kremers, et al. (2005b) revealed that cardiovascular disease was the primary cause of death in 49.7% of the patients. The authors discovered that the risk of cardiovascular death was higher among those RA patients who had at least 3 erythrocyte sedimentation rate values of greater or equal to 60 mm/hour, RA vasculitis, and RA-related lung disorders.

In a population-based analysis of trends over 40 years, Gabriel, et al. (2003) showed that RA disease complications, especially extraarticular manifestations of the disease and co-morbidities, are major factors in predicting the length of survival in this population.

A variety of other factors may affect survival patterns in RA patients. Maradit-Kremers, et al. (2005a) showed that these patients were less likely to report angina symptoms and were more likely to suffer unrecognized myocardial infarction and sudden cardiac death when compared to patients without RA.

Krishnan, et al. (2004) evaluated mortality from acute myocardial infarction among RA patients and found that mortality rates were higher in older patients and in men.

Osteoarthritis (OA)

Osteoarthritis (OA) is the most prevalent type of arthritis and is the leading cause of disability in older persons (Issa and Sharma, 2006; Managing Osteoarthritis, 3/14/2006). With the aging population increasing in the developed world, this disease will become more prevalent, and will require frequent treatment interventions (Franck, et al., 2005). Issa and Sharma (2006) have identified the following risk factors in the development of OA: aging; genetic factors; joint deformity and injury, and obesity and hormonal dysfunction. Schneider, et al. (2005), using the results of the First National Health Survey, in Germany, showed that age, obesity, and occupational stress conditions were correlates of OA.

In addition, Janssen and Mark (2006) analyzed data from the Third National Health and Nutrition Examination survey and discovered that body mass index predicted an increased risk of having arthritis and knee OA.

OA patients, like RA patients, are likely to have co-morbidities. In fact, OA has been described as the condition with the highest rate of co-morbidities (Caporali, et al., 2005). Schneider, et al. (2005)'s study revealed that OA patients had an increased likelihood of having osteoporosis, thyroid disorders, chronic bronchial disorders, hypertension, and high blood lipids. However, they did not have an elevated incidence of diabetes mellitus.

Using the results of the AMICA study in Italy, Caporali, et al. (2005) reported that the most prevalent co-morbidities among OA patients were hypertension, osteoporosis, type 2 diabetes (DM), chronic obstructive pulmonary disease, myocardial infarction, angina pectoris, and peptic ulcer disease. Other population-based research has shown that OA patients have an increased risk of developing peptic ulcer disease and renal disease (Gabriel, et al., 1999).

Older men with OA who already have co-morbid health problems may be at increased risk of developing additional co-morbid health problems. Gabriel, et al. (1999)'s study, used the Rochester Epidemiology Project, to determine that age, male gender, and baseline co-morbid health problems predicted an increased likelihood of co-morbidity. Caporali, et al. (2005)'s study in Italy also showed that co-morbidities were more prevalent in older OA patients.

Aging has been implicated as both as a risk factor in the development of the disease and as a condition that increases the progression of the condition (Issa and Sharma, 2006). Additional risk factors related to the worsening of the disease process include obesity, varus-valgus alignment, varus thrust, bone marrow edema lesions, and reduced hip abduction movement.

Inflammatory Arthritis (IA)

Inflammatory arthritis (IA) in the elderly has become a subject of interest to clinicians and investigators because of its frequency in older populations (Le Parc, 2005). Older individuals may develop syndromes that consist of rapid onset of the disease with pitting non-inflammatory edema. They may develop syndromes that are resistant to steroids, and thus are at increased risk for developing hemopathy or metastastic carcinoma. Various forms of mild seronegative arthritis in the elderly may be confused with polymyalgia rheumatism. In addition, some older men are at risk for developing late onset of inflammatory spondylarthropathy that presents as undifferentiated arthritis, fever, weight loss, and substantial edema.

Osteoporosis (OP)

The following conditions may increase the risk of osteoporotic (OP) fractures: calcium and vitamin D deficiencies; lack of physical activity; prolong immobilization, and the lack of fall prevention measures (Gass and Dawson-Hughes, 2006; Miazgowski, 2005).

Based on a sample of 425 community-dwelling individuals in Croatia, aged 50 years and older, Grazio, et al. (2005) showed that the prevalence of vertebral fractures increased with age. Other possible risk factors include hyperthyroidism, neuropsychiatric disorders and alcohol abuse (Gage, et al., 2006).

Wilkins and Birge (2005) suggest that problems with neuromuscular functioning that influences postural stability may more frequently contribute to OP fractures than problems associated with skeletal integrity. Iki, et al. (2006) also found that trunk muscle strength is a strong predictor of OP in postmenopausal women. Nevertheless, treating secondary causes of OP with drug therapies can help to prevent these fractures (Gass and Dawson-Hughes, 2006).

Researchers are evaluating the effects of free testosterone on bone mineral density (BMD) and prevalent fractures in elderly men. Based on the results of the MrOS study in Sweden, Mellstrom, et al. (2006) discovered that free testosterone is an independent predictor of reduced bone mineral density and prevalent fractures in a large cohort of elderly men.

Aged patients taking warfarin and other Vitamin K antagonists for the treatment of atrial fibrillation may be at increased risk of OP fractures (Gage, et al., 2006). Vitamin K helps to activate clotting factors and bone proteins, and warfarin impedes this process. Therefore, older persons taking warfarin on a long-term basis may be more vulnerable to OP fractures than those not taking the drug. Using data from the National Registry of Atrial Fibrillation, Gage, et al. (2006) showed that among men with atrial fibrillation, but not among women with this condition, taking warfarin on a long-term basis predicted OP fractures. Several factors were associated with a reduced risk of OP: African-American race, male gender, and treatment with beta-adrenergic antagonists. The investigators suggest that beta-adrenergic antagonists may protect against OP fractures.

Individuals with liver cirrhosis are also at risk for OP. Cijevschi, et al. (2005), using a sample of 150 patients with alcoholic or viral liver cirrhosis, discovered that 38% of the patients suffered from OP or osteopenia.

Researchers are also interested in factors that protect against OP. For example, Gage, et al. (2006) found that the following factors were related to a decreased risk of OP fractures: African-American race/ethnicity; male gender, and use of beta-adrenergic antagonists.

In addition to causing fractures, OP may increase the risk of cardiovascular disease in postmenopausal women. Based on a sample of 2,576 women with a mean age of 66.5 years, Tanko, et al. (2005) reported that women with OP were 3.9 times more likely to have cardiovascular events than women with higher bone mass. Their risk of cardiovascular incidents increased with the number and severity of baseline vertebral fractures.

Fibromyalgia (FM)

Fibromyalgia (FM) is a syndrome that is difficult to diagnose for it is characterized by widespread diffuse pain and tenderness at various specific anatomic sites. After ruling out other possible syndromes, FM has been diagnosed based on a classification criteria developed by the American College of Rheumatology. Such symptoms as tender point count, pain intensity, sleep disturbance, stiffness, headache, paresthesia, fatigue, irritable bowel syndrome, and sicca- and Raynaud-like symptoms have been used in making the diagnosis (Kozanoglu, et al., 2003; White, et al., 1999).

Using data from the London Fibromyalgia Epidemiology Study, White, et al. (1999) found that the most prevalent symptoms among persons with FM were musculoskeletal pain (77.3%), fatigue

(77.3%), severe fatigue lasting 24 hours after minimal activity (77%), non-restorative sleep (65.7%), and insomnia (56%).

Genetic, neuroendocrine, psychosocial, and traumatic factors have been considered as possible causes of the condition (Arnold, et al., 2004; Kozanoglu, et al., 2003). It is possible that FM is a secondary condition related to other diffuse pain syndromes (Gowin, 2000).

Infections may also be a factor in the development of FM. A case-control study by Kozanoglu, et al. (2003) found that when compared to a control group, hepatitis C infection patients had higher mean tender point count, pain intensity, sleep disorders, stiffness, paresthesia, and fatigue. However, these patients did not differ with controls in terms of irritable bowel syndrome and sicca- and Raynaud-like symptoms. The authors suggest that there may be a higher prevalence of FM in hepatitis C infection patients, and or that FM may develop in the progression of hepatitis C infection.

In addition, FM may be associated with thyroid autoimmunity. Ribeiro and Proietti (2004) used a case-control investigation to measure the possible relationship between FM and thyroid autoimmunity. The findings revealed that FM was associated with thyroid autoimmunity, which was based on the presence of detectable antithyroid peroxidase antibodies or antithyroglobulin antibodies. The association between FM and thyroid autoimmunity was increased even more after controlling for two confounding conditions, depression and age.

Low Back Pain (LBP)

D'Astolfo and Humphreys, 2006 claim that musculoskeletal pain, including low back pain (LBP), is one of the leading determinants of chronic health problems, in persons over 65 years of age. Back problems are also a common reason why aged adults see their health care practitioner (The American Geriatrics Society Foundation for Health in Aging, 2006).

Back problems in aged adults frequently differ from younger individuals. For example, younger people are more likely to suffer a slipped disk, while this is not likely to develop in adults older than 60 years (The American Geriatrics Society Foundation for Health in Aging, 2006). BP frequently becomes chronic in elder adults and often waxes and wanes. Among elder adults, neck pain is also prevalent. Tension in the neck muscles or spinal problems in the neck area often cause neck pain.

In elder adults, various conditions, such as cancer, infection, and degenerative spinal conditions can produce BP (The American Geriatrics Society Foundation for Health in Aging, 2006). Degenerative problems often result from wear and tear and include a narrowing along the spinal canal, lower spine instability, sciatica, and osteoporosis fractures.

Older adults are at risk for lumbar spinal stenosis or a narrowing within the lower part of the spinal canal (The American Geriatrics Society Foundation for Health in Aging, 2006). Bony growths that interfere or obstruct with the lower part of the spinal canal may cause this narrowing. These bony growths occur due to chronic wear, a protruding disk, or thickening of ligaments that are situated along the spine. As a result, individuals suffer from pain in their back or legs. The pain decreases when sitting, bending forward, walking uphill, or lying in a bent or flexed position and increases when standing or walking. Use of a cane or walker or other assistive device can reduce the pain.

Degenerative disk disease of the lower back over time may cause an individual's spine to become unstable (The American Geriatrics Society Foundation for Health in Aging, 2006). This occurs when a problem at one disk is out of proportion to the other disk spaces. This instability can push dome of the vertebrae forward, resulting in pinched spinal nerves and associated severe BP or severe pain down the back of the legs. A person often experiences this pain suddenly and it frequently occurs after a quick movement or extensive bending of the lower back. People with this condition can experience pain that lasts only minutes to hours. However, the pain often returns and with changes in a person's position.

Elder adults are susceptible to sciatica or pain and inflammation in the sciatic nerve (The American Geriatrics Society Foundation for Health in Aging, 2006). Sciatica often produces sharp pain that radiates from the buttock down the back of the leg to the foot. In other instances, the person feels the pain in one or two isolated locations within these anatomical areas.

Two prevalent patterns of sciatica occur in elder adults. In one pattern, the person feels the pain only when standing and walking (The American Geriatrics Society Foundation for Health in Aging,

2006). This pattern may restrict an individual's capacity to walk long distances. Pain occurs because of a narrowing along the lower spine. In the other pattern, persons may experience the pain suddenly when they are not moving. Their pain is exacerbated when they try to change their position suddenly. In several weeks, this sudden and constant pain often subsides spontaneously.

In aged adults, osteoporotic (OP) fractures of the backbones or vertebrae in the mid to lower back are a frequent cause of BP (The American Geriatrics Society Foundation for Health in Aging, 2006). In a study of residents at a long-term care facility, osteoporosis predicted chronic pain (D'Astolfo and Humphreys, 2006). OP thins the bone in the vertebrae, making them more susceptible to breaking. Persons who suffer an OP fracture may experience sudden pain, which is felt deep at the location of the fracture. However, the pain may also radiate to their side, abdomen, and legs and the area covering the involved vertebrae frequently feels very tender.

The pain resulting from a sudden vertebral fracture frequently has a duration ranging between two weeks and two months (The American Geriatrics Society Foundation for Health in Aging, 2006). The pain often becomes worse when an individual stands and walks and the pain is reduced when the person lies down. Individuals frequently have impairment in walking for about two weeks, and their activity is restricted for about a month.

In aged women, LBP may also result from osteoporosis and fractures in the lower area of the pelvis (The American Geriatrics Society Foundation for Health in Aging, 2006). These women usually experience sudden pain and it frequently involves the lower back. However, they can also experience pain in the buttocks or hip. In four to six weeks, the pain frequently subsides spontaneously. Women have a very good prognosis for recovery.

Back disorders can also be caused by other problems, such as certain cancers, infection in the backbones or spinal column, or an aneurysm (The American Geriatrics Society Foundation for Health in Aging, 2006). Persons older than 50 years, those with a history of cancer, and people with BP lasting longer than one month have an increased probability of having cancer as a cause of BP. Infection is more prevalent among individuals who are on hemodialysis, or who have an indwelling IV catheter, a history of urinary tract infections, and a history of intravenous drug abuse.

For persons with these conditions, the BP frequently becomes steadily worse over several to weeks and is not associated with being in any one position (The American Geriatrics Society Foundation for Health in Aging, 2006). These persons should contact a physician if they experience pain in the upper back, fever, pain radiating below the knee, problems walking, substantial pain after a fall, and loss of bowel or bladder control. Persons with known cancer who also develop back pain should be evaluated to determine if they have spinal cord problems.

Jacobs, et al. (2006) found that female gender was predictive of chronic back pain in persons aged 77 years. Based on a study of 489 individuals, aged 50-85 years, Tsuji, et al. (2001) also revealed that women were more likely than men to report low back pain.

Financial problems, feeling lonely, fatigue, poor self-reported health, dependence on help in activities of daily living (ADL), joint pain, and obesity have been found to be associated with chronic back pain (Jacobs, et al., 2006; Hartvigsen, et al., 2004). Other diseases such as OA have been predictive of back and neck pain (Hartvigsen, et al., 2004).

Disability and Quality of Life

Arthritis

With the aging of the United States population, it is expected that there will be an increase in the number of people with arthritis and its related disabilities and impaired quality of life (Hootman and Helmick, 2006). In addition, the epidemic of obesity with its negative effect on mobility will contribute to the disabling impact of arthritis.

Using the results of the National Health Interview Survey Disability Supplement Phase Two, Verbrugge and Juarez (2006) compared disabled arthritic adults to adults who were disabled due to other conditions. They found that those people with arthritis-associated impairments: 1. were less physically active, but were able to maintain social ties; 2. they had more impairments in all areas (e.g., self-care, managing a household, performing physical tasks) because of the pain and fatigue associated with their condition; 3. despite their disabilities, they relied on less assistance from other people, but used more equipment for assistance, and had more problems in moving around. The investigators suggest that more interventions should be developed for the home and workplace to enhance access and equipment for those with arthritis-associated disabilities.

Machado, et al. (2006) carried out a cross-sectional investigation of 1,606 older adults in Bambui, Brazil, to assess the effects of arthritis on disability and quality of life. They found that arthritis was correlated with having sleep problems, poor perceived health, impaired mobility, disability for a duration of two weeks, two physical disabilities, and two mental health problems.

In Stang, et al. (2006)'s study, arthritis predicted the inability to work or perform normal activities. However, co-morbid mental and physical health problems accounted for more than 50% of this association. Studies have shown that major predictors of disability in this population are depression, anxiety, cognitive impairment, and lower extremity arthritis (Sturnieks, et al., 2004).

Rheumatoid Arthritis (RA)

Allaire, et al. (2005) used data from the "National Data Bank for Rheumatic Diseases" and U.S. population figures to analyze the rate of work disability in adults, aged 55-64 years, who had RA. Their results indicated that these RA workers had lower rates of employment than persons of the same age in the general population despite the fact that the RA sufferers had higher levels of education. When compared to younger adults with RA, more of the project population was unemployed and more of them worked part time. However, the older employees used sick leave less, but had similar limitations in fulfilling job demands.

Researchers have examined the extent to which disability and quality of life vary depending on whether the older person has early-onset, or late RA (Pease, et al., 1999; Calvo-Alen, et al., 2005; Mikuls, et al., 2003). Based on a sample of 400 RA patients, Pease, et al. (1999) discovered that late-onset RA (disease onset at age 65 years or older) produces the same degree of adverse effects as in the early onset population.

Based on a study of 255 adult female RA patients (mean age 54.3 years), Orstavik, et al. (2005) found that patients with incident vertebral deformities were older, had lower bone mineral density, had higher disability, and more frequently had a prior non-vertebral fractures than patients without incident vertebral fractures.

Pain is prevalent among elder RA sufferers and increases with age and disease duration (Jakobsson and Hallberg, 2002).

Chronic pain in this population is linked to depression and associated impaired cognitive functioning, therefore inadequate pain management is another risk factor for disability (Sewell, 1998; Brown, et al., 2002).

In their study, Treharne, et al. (2005) showed that RA patients with co-morbid cardiovascular disease were older, more likely to be male, and less likely to be employed, and may have higher levels of depression than those without this problem.

Osteoarthritis (OA)

Osteoarthritis (OA) is the second leading cause of work disability in U.S. men over age 50 years and results in more hospitalizations annually than RA (Arden and Nevitt, 2006; Issa and Sharma, 2006). In addition to causing significant disability, the disease leads to impaired quality of life and diminished emotional well-being in older adults (Gass and Dawson-Hughes, 2006).

Risk factors associated with functional decline are similar to those associated with the progression of the disease (Felson, et al., 2000). Genetic predisposition, family history, female gender, and age are non-modifiable risk factors while other factors, including obesity and overweight, injury, quadriceps muscle strength, mis-alignment, and inflammatory or septic arthritis, can be modified and/or prevented.

The risk of disability in persons with OA is increased when the fol-lowing conditions are combined: 1) the disease itself, 2) inactivity, and 3) the aging process (March and Stenmark, 2001). A long period of inactivity increases the risk of disability that is exacerbated as the disease progresses. This problem is worsened by the societal belief that OA is just a "wear and tear" condition that is aggravated by exercise.

Obesity and overweight are associated with disability and reduced quality of life in this population because of their decreased mobility and the increased weight placed on their knees, which causes more pain and bone deterioration. This, in turn, lessens the OA person's ability to exercise which then lowers their chances of controlling their weight (Focht, et al., 2005).

Other factors involved in functional decline include lower per-ceived self-efficacy, laxity of the knee, reduced aerobic exercise, declining joint proprioception, and increased knee pain (Issa and Sharma, 2006).

The impact of OA on disability and quality of life may vary depending on the particular joint that is affected by the disease. When the larger joints, especially knee and hip joints, and/or the vertebral column are involved, disability will follow (Franck, et al., 2005). OA of these larger joints can interfere with one's ability to walk, cook, bathe, dress, use the toilet and perform household tasks (Managing Osteoarthritis, 3/14/2006). When afflicted joints are exercised infrequently, they begin to lose muscle tone, thus resulting in increasing disability.

In Italy, Cimmino, et al. (2005) evaluated the clinical presentation of OA of 17,567 women and 7,878 men in the AMICA study. They discovered that adults with OAs found hip pain to be more intrusive than their OA pain in the knee and hand.

Bookwala, et al. (2003), drew on a sample of 367 older persons with OA and showed that knee pain predicted decreased physical and social functioning, and increased depressive symptoms, plus poor self-reported health. The decreased social functioning then resulted in deeper depressive symptoms, lower self-reported health and so on in an ever increasing cycle. The investigators conclude that it is important to differentiate between social and physical functioning when evaluating OA pain.

Based on data from the AMICA study in Italy, Cimmino, et al. (2005) discovered that OA patients over 70 reported more intense pain than did younger OA patients.

There are possible gender differences in the experience of OA-associated pain. Cimmino, et al. (2005) showed that female patients reported more intense OA-related pain scores than male patients.

Osteoporosis (OP)

Osteoporotic (OP) fractures in aged populations are major determinants of pain, morbidity, disability, poor quality of life, and increased mortality risk (Cooper, et al., 2006; Hasserius, et al., 2005; O'Neill, et al., 2004). Based on a 12-year follow-up study in Sweden, Hasserius, et al. (2005) showed that women with vertebral fracture in the thoracic or lumbar spine had current back pain and reduced health status during the year before the 12-year follow-up. Women with a new vertebral fracture at the 12-year follow-up were more likely to have back pain during the year preceding the follow-up, compared to women who did not have a new fracture.

Findings from the Fracture Prevention Trial were used to evaluate the impact of new or worsening back pain in postmenopausal women with OP and previous vertebral fracture (Silverman, et al., 2005). The study revealed that 20.5% of the women who completed the Osteoporosis Assessment Questionnaire during all study periods had suffered new or worsening pain that resulted in poor physical functioning and emotional well-being.

Men and women with OP hip fractures are at risk for becoming disabled. Based on a case-control study of men with OP hip fractures, Pande, et al. (2006) found that men with OP hip fractures were apt to be disabled and have poor quality of life.

Based on a 1-year, prospective study of functional outcome and quality of life in elderly women following a hip fracture, Boonen, et al. (2004) found that 24% of the estimated functional decline was due to the hip fracture. Poor functional status at the time of hospital discharge was the best predictor of major disability and quality of life losses even though there was major recovery from the operation.

The severity of bone loss and the associated number of OP fractures may increase the risk of negative outcomes. In a study of ambulatory status of patients, aged 90 years and older, with hip fractures, Ishida, et al. (2005) showed that the greater the number of prevalent vertebral fractures, the poorer the recovery of the ability to walk. In addition, the authors reported that dementia diminished the patients' ability to regain ambulatory functioning.

Injurious falls lead to major disability and diminished quality of life. It is estimated that between 35 and 40% of persons older than 65 years suffer a fall, and that up to 5% of these falls result in fracture (Newton, et al., 2006).

Based on a sample of 408 consecutive patients older than 50 years who had fallen, Newton, et al. (2006) found that there was not an increased prevalence of OP among the women victims when compared to age-related norms. The authors suggest that initiating OP therapy empirically based solely on falls may be inappropriate.

Age increases disability and impairment of quality of life. Along with age, the increased prevalence of co-morbid health problems in older individuals with OP predicts future disability and diminished quality of life.

Fibromyalgia (FM)

The degree of disability and quality of life in elder persons with fibromyalgia (FM) vary depending on symptom severity, pain level and other conditions. One factor is whether the individuals with the condition are being seen in clinical settings. According to Wolfe, et al. (1995), persons with FM who are treated in clinics have a severe case of the disease, high pain levels, and considerable disability.

Age may be predictive of disability and quality of life in persons with FM. As noted previously, Cronan, et al. (2002) found that in older adults with the condition, symptom duration increased, but the intensity of the symptoms decreased. As a result, older individuals may be less impaired than younger persons. In Rustoen, et al. (2005)'s investigation, middle-aged Norwegian citizens were at higher risk for chronic pain than older aged Norwegians. In this study, older citizens had higher quality of life than the middle-aged.

Older disabled individuals with widespread musculoskeletal pain, including FM may be at increased risk for falls. Using data from a prospective population-based cohort investigation, Leveille, et al. (2002) showed that older disabled women with widespread musculoskeletal pain were at increased risk for falling during the follow-up period compared to those who had no pain or mild pain in one musculoskeletal site. Older disabled women with widespread pain also had an increased risk for recurring falls and fractures associated with these falls.

Low Back Pain (LBP)

Low back pain (LBP) is a major cause of self-reported poor health, disability, dependence in ADL (activities in daily living), decreased quality of life, and increased health care costs in older populations. Webb, et al. (2003) suggest that BP with associated disability continues to increase in older people. As the proportion of the aged in the developed world will increase significantly in future, disability and decreased quality of life in older adults with LBP will continue to be a major public health problem.

Using data from the Jerusalem Longitudinal Study, Jacobs, et al. (2006) found that chronic back pain was related to self-reported poor health, impaired functioning, dependence in ADL, and decreased quality of life. In their study, decreased quality of life consisted of such factors as feeling lonely and having financial problems.

Disability and quality of life in elder adults with LBP may vary depending on whether they are institutionalized or living in the community. According to D'Astolfo and Humphreys (2006), the profile of a resident with BP in an Ontario long-term care facility is female, has OP, is an independent or assisted walker, has mild to moderate dementia, and has low levels of depression.

The severity of disability in elder adults with LBP are influenced by a variety of factors such as associated back problems, e.g., disc degeneration, OP, OA, spinal stenosis, fractures, co-morbidity, coping strategies and resources, and level of social support.

Stress, Coping, and Social Support

Psychosocial Stress

Older arthritis sufferers can experience significant chronic pain, stress, depression, and other adverse health outcomes associated with the loss of their ability to function in every day activities (Tak, 2006; Tsai, et al., 2003; Penninx, et al., 1997). OA of the knee and hip joints is especially difficult for older adults because it impairs their ability to perform normal activities (Managing Osteoarthritis, 3/14/2006). Their joints become painful, stiff and swollen, leading to restricted motion, impaired physical functioning, decreased participation in social activities, and work disability. The combination of these factors can lead to substantial psychosocial stress and further impairs functional status.

Using a community-based study with 1,690 individuals, aged, 55-85 years, Penninx, et al. (1997) showed that arthritis sufferers had more symptoms of depression than those in the general population.

A qualitative study by Tak (2006) discovered that arthritis victims suffered stress in their daily lives that was associated with changes in their health status, inability to perform routine activities, prevalence of family problems, difficulties in managing finances, problems in their social interactions, and upheaval in their living situations.

Coping

Older individuals with arthritis use different strategies to cope with chronic pain and daily stressors (Tak, 2006). They: 1. use cognitive strategies, and participate in diversions to help them better understand and cope with chronic pain and the other stressors they face; 2. develop assertive strategies when interacting in social situations; 3. believe that they can control their environment; 4. have high levels of self-esteem (Penninx, et al., 1997).

Social Support

High-quality social support can be invaluable in helping arthritis sufferers function (Griffin, et al., 2001; Penninx, et al., 1997). Penninx, et al. (1997) revealed that having a partner, having numerous close social ties, and experiencing emotional support to report more severe RA symptoms over time and be rated by their rheumatologists as having increased disease status.

Treatment and Rehabilitation Outcomes

Rheumatoid Arthritis (RA)

Several studies have examined the role of nutrition in the development of inflammatory diseases such as rheumatoid arthritis (RA). Investigators in the European Prospective Investigation of Cancer (EPIC) Norfolk study have analyzed diet diaries from over 25,000 adults, aged, 45 to 74 year olds (University of Manchester, 2005). They followed these study subjects for a 9-year period to ascertain new incidents of inflammatory polyarthritis, including RA. Their findings indicated that individuals who eat more brightly-colored fruits and vegetables such as oranges, carrots and sweetcorn have a lower risk of developing rheumatoid arthritis and other forms of inflammatory polyarthritis. Brightly-colored fruit and vegetables contain vitamin C and the pigment, beta-cryptoxanthin, which may serve as antioxidants that protect against inflammation producing oxidative damage. The authors in the EPIC Norfolk study found that in 88 patients who acquired inflammatory polyarthritis, their average daily intake of beta-cryptoxanthin was 40% lower than in persons who did not develop this disease. The study participants who developed inflammatory polyarthritis had a 20% lower average intake of another carotenoid, zeaxanthin than those who did not develop inflammatory polyarthritis. Individuals in the study who were in the top third of beta-cryptoxanthin intake were only 50% as likely to acquire inflammatory polyarthritis as those in the lowest third. In addition, vitamin C intake was associated with a reduced risk of developing inflammatory polyarthritis. Other research has shown that eating large amounts of red meat is related to an increased risk of inflammatory polyarthritis (University of Manchester, 2005).

Nonsteroidal anti-inflammatory drugs can help relieve pain for RA patients. However, these medications do not treat the disease progression. Standard treatment for the disease consists of medications that suppress the immune system and can modify disease progression (Stanford University Medical Center, 2005). These medications are known as disease modifying anti-rheumatic drugs (DMARDs), and methotrexate is the most frequently used drug in this category (Center for the Advancement of Health, 2005). Methotrexate originally was designed as a treatment for cancer. Only one DMARD, leflunomide, was designed as a treatment for RA. Researchers are evaluating new therapies to help the many RA sufferers who do not get pain relief and control of their disease with existing treatments.

In recent years, new drugs have been created that block the immune system's response and, these drugs known as TNF (tumor necrosis factor) blockers. These medications prevent TNF from signaling the release of substances that damage joints. Two such TNF blockers are etanercept (Enbrel) and infliximab (Remicade).

Schiff, et al. (2006) investigated the effects of long-term RA treatment with etanercept for patients 65 years and older and those under 65 years. Functional disability was measured using the Health Assessment Questionnaire-Disability Index. Their results, based on multiple controlled and open-label extension trials, showed that both age groups when treated with etanercept had similar and quick enhancement in function.

With the aging of the population, the costs of different RA treatments have become particularly critical. One retrospective study by Weycker, et al. (2005) compared the costs of etanercept with infliximab during the first year of treatment in a sample of RA patients age 65 years and older. Using two large, automated health care claims databases in the U.S., the researchers discovered that the mean total cost of treating patients with etanercept was lower than for patients treated with infliximab ($12,159 vs. $22,347).

The use of infliximab and other anti-TNF-alpha blockades may enhance insulin resistance in RA patients thus putting them at risk for developing cardiovascular disease because the insulin resistance promotes endothelial dysfunction. It is theorized that a TNF-alpha blockade may reduce insulin serum levels and enhance insulin resistance in patients who have not responded to conventional treatments.

Gonzalez-Gay, et al. (2006), using a sample of 27 rheumatoid arthritis patients in Spain, evaluated the impact of infliximab infusion on insulin resistance. The results of their study showed that infliximab rapidly improved insulin resistance and insulin sensitivity in RA patients. The authors suggest that anti-TNF-alpha blockades may be beneficial for long-term use since they may fight against the development of atherosclerosis.

The FDA has approved the biologic drug, adalimumab (Humira) for treating adults with moderate to severe RA who do not well with other therapies (Center for the Advancement of Health, 2005). Adalimumab works as a TNF blocker. It prevents TNF from signaling the release of substances that damage joints.

A review of the clinical literature found that the combination of adalimumab (Humira) with methotrexate is about five times more efficacious than methotrexate by itself (Center for the Advancement of Health, 2005). Based on six randomized controlled trials involving 2,381 individuals who had the disease for at least 10 years, adalimumab, combined with methotrexate, reduced pain and swelling in those patients who had been treated unsuccessfully with conventional therapies. Forty-three percent of all of the patients receiving the combination of adalimumab and methotrexate had attained 50% reduction of their symptoms, while only 9% of all the participants had achieved this level after being on a combination of placebo and methotrexate.

Some researchers are focusing their efforts on new drugs that work on mechanisms that activate T cells, which are immune cells considered important in the etiology of RA (Stanford University Medical Center, 2005). Abatacept is the first of a class of drugs known as co-stimulation modulators, which selectively block one of the two signals that are necessary to trigger T cells. The drug may be useful in treating RA patients who do not respond to standard treatments.

Genovese, et al. (2005) evaluated the effectiveness and safety of abatacept using a randomized, double-blind, phase-three trial. Study participants were patients with active RA who had not responded adequately to anti-TNF-alpha treatment for at least three months. The investigators used the American College of Rheumatology standard, 20% or greater improvement in functional impairment. Functional impairment was measured using the Health Assessment Questionnaire evaluation of disability. The results showed that at a six months follow-up, more patients who were treated with abatacept showed greater enhancement in functional ability than patients in the placebo group. The incidence of adverse side effects was similar in both the treatment and placebo groups.

Based on a double-blind, placebo-controlled clinical trial involving 339 RA patients, Emery, et al. (2006a) evaluated the impact of combining abatacept with methotrexate on health-related quality of life. The researchers used the SF-36 Health Survey to measure changes in health-related quality of life. The findings indicated that after 12 months of treatment, patients in the abatacept group (10 mg/kg) combined with methotrexate had better overall health-related quality of life compared to patients in the placebo plus methotrexate group.

Drugs that are designed to suppress inflammation-causing cytokines, especially those associated with T cells, have enhanced RA therapy. However, remissions attained by these biologic treatments are below 50% (eMaxHealth, 2006). Investigators have targeted B cells to enhance the remission rates of biologic treatments. For example, researchers are evaluating the biologic agent, rituximab, which selectively reduces the amount of B cells.

The efficacy and safety of rituximab plus methotrexate in patients with active RA has been assessed. Using a sample of 465 patients with active rheumatoid arthritis who have been resistant to DMARDs, Emery, et al. (2006b) found that two rituximab doses (500 mg and 1,000 mg when added to methotrexate were efficacious and tolerated well.

Osteoarthritis (OA)

Drugs are intended to relieve pain in osteoarthritis patients. Research has revealed that acetaminophen up to 4,000 milligrams is the choice of medications for elder OA patients. Acetaminophen use has limited adverse complications but can include liver toxicity associated with fasting or substantial alcohol use and kidney failure due to long-term use of the drug (Hochberg, et al., 1995a; Griffin, et al., 1995).

If pain persists, non-steroidal, anti-inflammatory drugs (NSAIDs) can be prescribed (Hochberg, 1995a; Hochberg, 1995b; Griffin, et al., 1995). However, research has indicated that NSAIDs offer little pain relief or enhancement in functional status and are associated with ulcers, bleeding, and gastrointestinal perforation. Studies have shown that elder patients who take NSAIDs have higher rate of emergency and hospital services than non-users, and this increases health care costs (Managing Osteoarthritis, 3/14/2006; Smalley, et al., 1996). For example, an investigation of Medicaid recipients, aged 65 years and older, found that users of NSAIDs were more likely to be hospitalized and use the emergency department than non-users (Smalley, et al., 1996).

There have been attempts to alter health care providers' treatment strategies to substitute acetaminophen for NSAID. Stein and Griffin (2001) evaluated the impact of an educational program for nursing home physicians and nursing staff to achieve this goal. Physicians and nursing staff in the study participated in an educational program about the appropriate treatment for muscle and joint pain and were asked to substitute acetaminophen for NSAID therapy in all nursing home patients, aged 65 years and older. If their patients did not improve with acetaminophen, the clinicians could add ibuprofen to their regimen. If this treatment was not effective, the providers could return to prescribing regular NSAID treatment. The results of the investigation showed that acetaminophen use increased from an average of two days per week to five days per week, while NSAID use was reduced from seven days a week to less than two days per week. The patients did not report any substantial increase in pain or disability.

The use of opioids has been shown to be useful for short-term amelioration of acute worsening of pain. However, older patients may have trouble tolerating codeine as a long-term regimen (Hochberg, et al., 1995a; Griffin, et al., 1995).

Patients with knee OA for whom oral analgesics are not effective or desirable may be treated with capsaicin cream or other topical treatment (Hochberg, et al., 1995b; Puett and Griffin, 1994; Griffin, et al., 1995). For patients who have swelling and inflammation in their knees, injections of corticosteroid into the joint have been found to be useful (Holman and Lorig, 1997; Hochberg, et al., 1995b). However, they are not recommended for patients with hip OA because repeated injections results in progressive damage of cartilage (Hochberg, et al., 1995a).

Hyalgan is the first FDA-approved hyaluronan therapy for OA knee pain. It is indicated for OA of the knee in patients who have failed to respond to conservative non-pharmacologic treatment and to simple analgesics. Hyalgan, a compound made from roosters' combs, is injected in OA knees and can give 6 months of pain relief. Incremental improvement in pain relief has been obtained with repeat treatment cycles.

Ganz, et al. (2006), using a sample of 339 OA patients, measured the effectiveness of care and the level of safety associated with the provision of treatment. The investigators discovered that the quality of OA treatment was deficient, especially in terms of medication safety. They recommended more appropriate use of medications, advising patients about their use of medications, and making better use of effective OA regimens.

Surgery is recommended for patients with knee osteoarthritis if they do not respond to medical treatment. OA patients may obtain relief from their pain and improve their functioning with surgical repair and replacement of their knee joints (Hochberg, et al., 1995b; Wright, et al., 1995). However, aged persons should be aware of the possibility of surgical complications. Simultaneous surgery on both knees is discouraged, but remains the surgeons' and patients' decisions.

Occupational therapy can help OA patients minimize their pain and improve their physical, social, and emotional functioning. These therapists assess a person's ability to participate in activities of daily living and recommend modifications needed, such as elevated toilet seats or wall bars in bathtubs. They teach patients how to protect their joints and conserve energy and may recommend living on one floor of a residence to help the patient avoid pain by not climbing steps, kneeling or squatting (Managing Osteoarthritis, 3/14/2006; Hochberg, et al., 1995a; Hochberg, et al., 1995b).

Various investigations have studied the effects of occupational therapy in minimizing disability in older patients with osteoarthritis (Managing Osteoarthritis, 3/14/2006; Clark, et al., 1997). In the Well Elderly Study, Clark, et al. (1997) studied the impact of occupational therapy in helping persons, aged 60 and older, avoid disability over a 9-month period. The experimental group received occupational therapy that emphasized joint protection, adaptive equipment, safety at home and in the community, exercise, conserving energy, nutrition, and other issues. The control group participated in a program that only dealt with dances, games, and other social activities. The findings revealed that individuals who participated in the occupational therapy had better social interactions, less, pain, improved health, greater satisfaction with life and better functional status. Six months after the study period, participants in the occupational therapy continued to report improved outcomes.

Osteoporosis (OP)

Prevention is the primary treatment for osteoporosis (OP), and is aimed at reducing bone loss and minimizing fracture risk (American Geriatrics Society Foundation for Health in Aging, 2006). Prevention consists of identifying and reducing the risk factors by appropriate testing of BMD and recommending appropriate exercise and nutrition.

Individuals who participate in moderate to vigorous exercise at least three times per week can increase bone mass and reduce the risk of fractures (American Geriatrics Society Foundation for Health in Aging, 2006). Walking and other weight-bearing exercises are the best forms of physical activity. Strength training, such as lifting weights and other types of resistance training enhances the strength of hip bones and minimizes the risks of injurious falls and fractures. Strength training is also beneficial for muscle mass, strength, and balance in postmenopausal women.

Persons who are bed-bound or experience other types of severe reduction in physical activity can suffer significant bone mass. As a result, it is essential to return to regular physical activity as soon as possible after any disabling condition such as a stroke or a hospitalization (American Geriatrics Society Foundation for Health in Aging, 2006).

In terms of nutrition, persons 65 years and older and younger postmenopausal women should have a daily calcium intake of a minimum of 1,200 mg (American Geriatrics Society Foundation for Health in Aging, 2006). This requirement can be met by consuming calcium-rich foods, such a dairy products, eggs, and broccoli, taking calcium supplements and drinking calcium-fortified fruit juices. Calcium supplements are especially critical for postmenopausal women in the U.S. since their average daily calcium intake is 500-700 mg.

Researchers are analyzing the impact of calcium supplements on preventing fractures and bone structure in elder persons. A 5-year population-based clinical trial involving 1,460 women, older than 70 years, found that 56.8% of the patients who took 80% or more of their calcium supplements annually were less likely to have a fracture, compared to patients in the placebo group who took a comparable percentage of "dummy" pills (Prince, et al., 2006). Patients who took calcium supplements were also more likely to have improved bone structure when compared to patients in the placebo group. The authors conclude that calcium supplements are not effective in preventing clinical fractures in the aged population due to low compliance on a long-term basis. However, it is effective in patients who are compliant.

In addition, aged persons should have between 400 and 800 IU of vitamin D on a daily basis (American Geriatrics Society Foundation for Health in Aging, 2006). These individuals can obtain vitamin D in milk, fortified fruit juices, and other food. Vitamin D is also formed in the skin as a result of direct sunlight exposure. However, with the aging process, vitamin D production is less efficiently produced by sunlight. Therefore, all adults should take a daily supplement of a minimum of 400 IU of vitamin D, which are found in most multivitamins.

A 2-year randomized controlled trial evaluated the effects of reduced fat calcium- and vitamin D3-fortified milk on bone loss at clinically relevant skeletal sites vulnerable for fracture risk in 149 men over age 50 years (Daly, et al., 2006). The study evaluated whether supplements with calcium/vitamin D3-fortified milk giving an additional 1,000 mg of calcium and 800 IU of Vitamin D3, daily suppressed parathyroid hormone (PTH) and prevented or slowed bone loss at important skeletal sites. The findings of the trial revealed that after two years, BMD change was less at several skeletal sites in patients receiving the supplements compared to patients in the control group. Patients in the intervention group had an increase in serum 25 (OH) D and a decrease in PTH compared to patients in the control group.

Persons who smoke cigarettes and abuse alcohol are also at increased risk for OP (American Geriatrics Society Foundation for Health in Aging, 2006). Smoking cessation and limiting alcohol intake significantly reduces OP risks and also reduces the risk of cancer, cardiovascular disease, and lung disease.

Besides preventing the disease through exercise, dietary calcium intake, and modifying alcohol and cigarette smoking habits, certain drugs can help treat OP. In addition, specific medications are designed to increase bone mass. These include alendronate, raloxifene, risedronate, and ibandronate (American Geriatrics Society Foundation for Health in Aging, 2006). These medications are taken to prevent OP in women who are at high risk for the disease. They are also used to reduce fracture risk in high-risk women who have OP.

Studies have been underway to evaluate which are the most effective treatments for reducing the risk of OP fractures. Bisphosphonates (e.g., alendronate, risedronate, and ibandronate) have been assessed for their long-term efficacy and safety (Epstein, 2006; Iwamoto, et al., 2006). Based on a review of articles between August 1985 and August 2005, Epstein (2006) found that bisphosphonates seem to offer the best antiresorptive effectiveness. Some bisphosphonates have been shown to produce 7% to 8% increase in BMD and 60% to 70% reduction in bone resorption markers. In terms of treating fracture risks, Epstein (2006) concludes that bisphosphonates may reduce new vertebral fracture incidence by 50% to 52%. The author concludes that at the present time bisphosphonates are the first-line treatments for OP. The author also notes that intermittent regimens of the newer bisphosphonates hold promise for being a better alternative to daily administration of the medication.

In their review of the literature, Iwamoto, et al. (2006) found that the bisphosphonates, alendronate and risedronate, prevent hip fractures. Alendronate and risedronate is viewed as first-line treatments for older women with OP who have risk factors for falls. Clinical trials have shown that the incidence of gastrointestinal problems between postmenopausal women with OP treated with bisphophonates and those in control groups are similar. Moreover, the long-term effectiveness and safety of alendronate and risedronate in treating OP in postmenopausal women have been demonstrated.

After reviewing the recent literature, Iwamoto, et al. (2006) reports that raloxifene, calcitonin, PTH, and strontium ranelate are effective in preventing vertebral fractures in postmenopausal women with OP. Raloxifene may be used in treating postmenopausal women with mild OP or osteopenia since it has been found to be efficacious in preventing initial vertebral fractures in these women. PTH and strontium have been shown to be effective in preventing non-vertebral fractures. However, PTH has been used in treating OP for two years or less. Other anti-resorptive drugs may be used after completing PTH therapy since this will help maintain the skeletal effects obtained during the PTH treatment.

Seeman (2006) reviewed the data on the effectiveness of strontium ranelate in reducing the risk of vertebral and non-vertebral fractures. The Treatment of Peripheral Osteoporosis study assessed the impact of strontium ranelate on non-vertebral fractures, and found that the drug reduced the risk of fractures in this population. A new drug, lasofoxifene, has also been evaluated for its effectiveness in preventing bone loss. Based on a randomized controlled study, McClung, et al. (2006) compared the effects of lasofoxifene with raloxifene and placebo in preventing bone loss in 410 postmenopausal women, aged 47 to 74 years. Their results indicated that women treated with either lasofoxifene (0.25 mg/day or 0.25 mg/day or 1.0 mg/day) were more likely to have increased their lumbar spine BMD than those treated with raloxifene or placebo. The incidence of adverse events was similar in both lasofoxifene and raloxifene and those treated with both drugs had low rates of discontinuations associated with adverse events. The investigators conclude that lasofoxifene may be an effective and safe therapy for preventing bone loss in postmenopausal women.

Estrogen/progesterone replacement therapy has been undertaken to prevent osteoporosis. However, this therapy should not be the first-line treatment because some types of estrogen treatment have increased the risks of breast cancer, cardiovascular disease, and deep-vein thrombosis (American Geriatrics Society Foundation for Health in Aging, 2006).

Efforts have been underway to assess the cost-effectiveness of medical treatments. Based on a cohort study of OP women, aged 65 years or older, Pfister, et al. (2006) evaluated the cost-effectiveness of several medications: calcitonin, raloxifene, bisphosphates, and PTH. Their study indicated that bisphosphonates was the only cost-effective medication to prevent fractures.

Treatment of fractures has been managed by standard medical or surgical interventions (American Geriatrics Society Foundation for Health in Aging, 2006). A more recent treatment option for spinal vertebrae fractures includes vertebroplasty. This procedure consists of injecting bone cement into the collapsed vertebrae. Another newer treatment, kyphoplasty, involves placing a balloon into the fractured vertebrae. Initial research suggests that these procedures can reduce pain, enhance functioning, and improve quality of life.

Anti-inflammatory medications and narcotics are used to control fracture-related pain (American Geriatrics Society Foundation for Health in Aging, 2006). Acute and chronic pain is also managed by physical therapy. Pain management involves the use of postural exercises and alternative techniques. Moreover, physical therapists provide recommendations of changing body mechanics, which can help prevent subsequent fractures.

A number of studies have found deficiencies in the treatment of OP after fragility fracture (Giangregorio, et al., 2006; Feldstein, et al., 2006). Giangregorio, et al. (2006) conducted a systematic review of articles from 1996 to February 2005 to describe the treatment of OP following fragility fracture. Based on a sample of 35 studies, the authors discovered that there is inadequate treatment following a fragility fracture. Between 2 and 62% of the patients in the studies reported using calcium/vitamin D and between 1 and 65% reported taking OP medications. Physicians were more likely to recommend that women receive OP treatment than men. Patients with vertebral fractures were more like to get therapy than those with non-vertebral fractures. Physicians were more likely to diagnose older patients with the disease than younger patients. However, younger patients were more likely to get treatment than older patients.

The results of their investigation also showed that between 7 and 67% of the patients had a history of fracture and between 1 and 22% of the patients suffered a new fracture during the follow-up period (Giangregorio, et al., 2006). The authors found that fall assessments frequently were not reported, and when fall assessments were reported, they had been done infrequently.

Communication about at-risk patients to physicians may be helpful in improving the treatment of patients who are at risk for OP fracture. Based on a prospective cohort study of 111 aged persons in assisted living facilities, Setter, et al. (2005) assessed the efficacy of an intervention consisting of communicating OP evaluation and fracture risk to physicians. The investigators evaluated the fracture risk in a female cohort with no known prior OP diagnosis and discovered that they had a high risk of suffering a fracture over the next 5 years. The findings also revealed that there was increased use of OP treatments when the patients' physicians received a communication about the patients' OP assessment and fracture risk. For example, in the intervention group, there was an increase in the percentage of patients who started using calcium or vitamin D supplements. In the intervention group, 8 patients also started using bisphosphonates. In contrast, there were no significant increases in OP therapy in the control group. However, communication to physicians did not result in an increase in the percentage of patients obtaining a BMD evaluation.

Another study of clinician communication evaluated the efficacy of electronic medical record reminders in improving management of OP after a fracture (Feldstein, et al., 2006). Based on a sample of 311 female patients, aged 50 to 89 years, who had suffered a fracture but had not received a BMD evaluation or OP drugs, Feldstein, et al. (2006) discovered that 51.5% of patients received a BMD evaluation or OP drugs when their providers received a electronic medical record reminder, compared to only 5.9% of the patients who were in the usual care group. The authors conclude that electronic medical record reminders could enhance OP treatment for persons suffering fractures as electronic medical records are implemented in more clinical settings. The researchers recommend further research into the possible barriers to and opportunities for improving the care of post-fracture OP patients.

Fibromyalgia (FM)

Evidence about the effectiveness of FM treatment is lacking. Clinical trials have been limited because of methodological problems, such as short duration and the lack of masking (Goldenberg, et al., 2004). The FDA has not approved any specific medical treatment for FM.

Despite the weaknesses in clinical research, some treatments have been found to have some clinical effectiveness for FM patients (Goldenberg, et al., 2004). According to a review of clinical trials, low-dose tricyclic antidepressants, cardiovascular exercise, cognitive-behavioral therapy, and patient education have been shown to have some benefits (Goldenberg, et al., 2004).

Recent research has evaluated the effectiveness of pregabalin, a alpha (2)-delta ligand for the treatment of FM (Crofford, et al., 2005). This drug has been found to be a safe and effective treatment for neuropathic pain (related to diabetic neuropathy and post-herpetic neuralgia), epilepsy, and anxiety (Shneker and McAuley, 2005; Zareba, 2005). Using a multi-center, double-blind study of 529 FM patients, Crofford, et al. (2005) evaluated the effects of pregabalin on pain, sleep, and health-related quality of life. They discovered that pregabalin at 450 mg per day was effective in treating FM-associated pain symptoms, sleep problems, and fatigue, compared to a placebo. The most common adverse events were dizziness and sleepiness.

In contrast, trigger point injections and other commonly used FM treatments have not been found to have positive effects. Research suggests that a stepwise approach focusing on education, exercise, cognitive-behavioral treatment, low-dose tricyclic antidepressants, or all four approaches should be followed. Therapy should emphasize both symptom relief and modifying the patients' perceptions of their condition and assisting them in developing effective coping behaviors. Clinicians should be aware of the possible adverse effects of low-dose tricyclic antidepressants for older patients who may be especially sensitive to these medications and have counter-indications because they are taking other medications (http://www.drkoop.com/ency/93/guides/000076_7.html).

Treatment approaches should be individualized, taking into account the older patients' physical and psychosocial functioning (http://www.drkoop.com/ency/93/guides/000076_7.html). Patients should undertake all therapies with the belief that the treatments are trial and error since there is no clear treatment available. Patients and clinicians should work together to make the best decisions given the patients' symptoms and preferences. Patients should be aware that their treatments may be life long and should not be discouraged by relapses. Improve in FM symptoms is subjective. Some patients are satisfied with only a 10% reduction in their symptoms. It is also important to involve family and friends in the management of the patients' symptoms, especially in cardiovascular exercise activities. In addition, participation in FM support groups may be beneficial for patients and their family and friends.

Initially, FM patients may treat their symptoms with physical therapy, exercise, stress management, and cognitive-behavioral treatment (http://www.drkoop.com/ency/93/guides/000076_7.html). If these non-medication approaches fail to alleviate symptoms, low-dose tricyclic antidepressants can be added to the patients' treatment.

Low-dose tricyclic antidepressants have a positive impact on the central nervous system by improving pain tolerance. These medications cause drowsiness which can be helpful to FM patients who often have difficulty sleeping. In addition, patients can benefit from participating in patient education programs which help them to enhance their coping skills.

Therapy should also focus on treating syndromes associated with the condition. FM-associated syndromes include cognitive impairment, chronic fatigue, restless leg syndrome, multiple sensitivities, irritable bowel syndrome, irritable bladder syndrome, and neurally-mediated hypotension.

Low Back Pain (LBP) Treatment

Basic treatment for low back pain (LBP) is rest and pain relievers since LBP often causes muscle spasms (American Geriatrics Society Foundation for Health in Aging, 2006). Additional medical evaluation should be performed if the pain does not subside in a few weeks. LBP caused by infections, cancer, or aneurysms should be treated by treating the underlying condition.

Physical therapy may also be helpful for older adults with LBP. Physical therapy includes stretching, strengthening and pain relief exercises, and low-impact aerobic conditioning (Diabetic-Lifestyle. com,http://www.diabetic-lifestyle.com/articles/nov99_burni_1. htm). A gentle exercise program can be initiated after the initial symptoms have been reduced (American Geriatrics Society Foundation for Health in Aging, 2006). This exercise program can increase the strength in the back and stomach muscles, resulting in increased spinal stability. A water exercise program is the best technique because it provides for quick rehabilitation and the probability of re-injuring the back is low. Two simple water exercises are walking in chest-high water and doing the flutter kick. Back braces are also helpful in keeping the lower spine immobile.

Surgery may be indicated for severely pinched nerves. However, surgery does not always produce positive results. For persistent pain due to spinal instability, it may be necessary to perform surgery to fuse vertebrae together. This operation can restrict motion and reduce the instability and associated pain. Surgeries, such as a laminectomy, which relieve pressure on the spinal cord and stabilize the spine are beneficial for aged adults with lumbar spinal stenosis.

Vertebroplasty is a fairly new treatment for OP vertebral fractures. This surgery involves injecting cement into the collapsed vertebrae (American Geriatrics Society Foundation for Health in Aging, 2006). However, we still do not know the long-term outcome of this surgery.

Studies have shown that acupuncture, corticosteroid injection and other less traditional treatments have not been demonstrated to be beneficial on a consistent basis (American Geriatrics Society Foundation for Health in Aging, 2006). However, research continues to assess the effectiveness of percutaneous electrical nerve stimulation (PENS), also known as electrical acupuncture, and other less traditional treatments in aged adults (ClinicalTrials.gov, http://www.clinicaltrials.gov/show/NCT00101387). Researchers are also investigating the effects of certain surgical procedures, such as the lumbar total disc arthroplasty, in patients older than 60 years of age with disabling LBP (Bertagnoli, et al., 2006). More research is needed to assess outcomes for patients in this age group.

In terms of standard treatment, research has shown some deficits in the analgesic treatment of older people for LBP and other pain symptoms in geriatric care settings (Lovheim, et al., 2006; McClean and Higginbotham, 2002). Under-treatment of pain in aged adults is a prevalent problem. Lovheim (2006) evaluated pain prevalence and geriatric staff awareness of analgesic treatment for their residents based on a cross-sectional study of all geriatric care units in the county of Vasterbotten, Sweden. The results showed that 56.7% of the sample reported being in pain. Of those residents reporting pain, 27.9% did not receive any analgesics on a regular basis. Staff members who knew the resident best thought that the resident was receiving analgesic treatment in 72.7% of the cases in which residents reported being in pain but had no pharmacological treatment. The investigators recommend better communication among geriatric care staff to minimize the problem of under-treatment of pain in geriatric residents.

Engle, et al. (2001) compared the accuracy and bias of licensed practical nurse (LPN) and nursing assistant (NA) ratings of pain in a sample of 252 nursing home residents. They found that both LPNs and NAs underestimated the pain frequency and pain intensity of nursing home residents. NAs were found to be more accurate than LPNs in rating pain intensity. The findings also revealed that nursing home resident characteristics, e.g., race, gender, mental status, did not bias the pain ratings by either the LPNs or the NAs.

Patient Education and Self-Management

Older adults with OA may not always adhere to their pain regimen. They may be less likely to take pain medications compared to other prescribed medications. Using interviews with older adults in Toronto with disabling hip and knee OA, Sale, et al. (2006) evaluated adherence to pain regimen. Most of the participants in their in-depth, qualitative study had co-morbid conditions (e.g., DM and cardiovascular disease), and they were taking prescription medications for these diseases. The interviews revealed that the OA sufferers felt reluctant to take their prescription pain medications for OA compared to their prescription medications for their other diseases. The individuals with arthritis, when taking their prescription medications, tended to take them at lower doses or less frequency than prescribed. These persons, who had physical disabilities, nevertheless minimized their pain severity and reported a high tolerance for pain. They felt that other arthritis sufferers are treated appropriately and adhere to pain regimens.

Aged persons suffering from OP may also have difficulties in complying with their medication regimen. Patients may discontinue treatment because of adverse gastrointestinal events and other problems. Patients frequently stop therapy with bisphosphonates although they have been shown to be efficacious in treating osteoporosis (Penning-van Beest, et al. (2006). Based on a study of 2,124 women, aged 55 years and older, in The Netherlands, Penning-van Beest, et al. (2006) evaluated determinants of persistence with these drugs. The investigators discovered that patients taking alendronate weekly were more likely to continue with treatment than those who took the medication daily. Those patients who took risedronate, etidronate, and alendronate on a daily basis have similar rates of persistence with the drugs. Moreover, patients who suffered adverse gastrointestinal events after taking the medications were less likely to continue with these drugs. The authors conclude that dose interval and incidence of adverse gastrointestinal events were independent predictors of continuation with bisphosphonate treatment. Rates of continuation were still sub-optimal even though the rates were higher in patients who used the medications less frequently.

Solomon, et al. (2005) note that asymptomatic individuals may not take their medications regularly. Treatment compliance is especially critical for OP sufferers who are at risk for fractures.

Solomon, et al. (2005) evaluated compliance with OP medications using a retrospective cohort study of 40,002 Medicare patients. The investigators evaluated Medicare patients who began use of alendronate sodium, calcitonin, hormone therapy, raloxifene hydrochloride, or risedronate between January 1, 1998 and December 31, 2002. They discovered 45.2% of the Medicare patients were not continuing to fill their OP prescriptions one year after starting to take OP medications. About 52% of the patients were not continuing to fill their OP prescriptions five years after going on osteoporosis drugs.

To enhance older patients' compliance with their regimens, it is necessary to determine their use of dietary and health supplements. To what extent are these individuals following their medical regimens as well as taking dietary and health supplements? To what extent are certain persons taking dietary and health supplements instead of their prescribed treatments? More research is needed to assess predictors of dietary and health supplements. Brownie (2006) conducted a survey of about 1,200 randomly selected Australians, aged 65 to 98 years, to determine correlates of dietary and health supplement use. The findings of the survey revealed that female gender, arthritis, OP, back problems, and other chronic musculoskeletal problems predicted increased use of dietary and health supplements. Brownie (2006) suggests that older persons who use supplements may believe that supplements help relieve their chronic pain.

Aged arthritis sufferers can obtain better health outcomes if they receive education and training about their disease since this helps them to become active participants in their own care (Managing Osteoarthritis, 3/14/2006). Effective clinician-patient relationships are essential for managing arthritis.

In terms of OA self-management, an effective clinician-patient relationship can facilitate appropriate use of medications, encourage behavioral change, help patients interpret and report symptoms of OA, cope with psychosocial stress, and help patients participate in treatment decisions (Managing Osteoarthritis, 3/14/2006). Clinicians must learn to work with patients as partners to achieve these goals. Telephone support from clinician offices can be especially helpful in helping patients modify their behaviors and cope with symptoms and do not significantly increase health care costs for either clinicians or patients (Hochberg, et al., 1995a; Managing Osteoarthritis, 3/14/2006). Clinicians can use telephone conversations with patients to discuss patients' problems with joint pain, medication (type, dosage, and toxicities), treatment adherence, and barriers to obtaining care.

Studies have demonstrated that patient education programs are particularly helpful in achieving positive health care outcomes by providing OA patients with the knowledge and skills necessary for self-management. For example, the Chronic Disease Self-Management Program has been shown to be effective in helping OA patients interpret and report symptoms reliably and have reduced pain feelings of depression, and health care service utilization in chronic disease patients (Holman and Lorig, 1997; Managing Osteoarthritis, 3/14/2006; Agency for Healthcare Research and Quality, 2002).

Various community-based organizations offer a range of services to help elder OA patients in their self-management activities. Self-help programs, support groups, exercise, informational meetings, and mobile services for transportation and meals are available for some aged OA sufferers.

Modifying older patients' behaviors, e.g., getting them to perform regular physical activity and altering how they perceive OA symptoms have been shown to improve symptoms or slow the progression of the disease (Holman and Lorig, 1997; Managing Osteoarthritis, 3/14/2006). Regular physical activity has a number of major benefits for elder OA patients. It can reduce arthritis pain, enhance functional status, and delay the onset of disability (Shih, et al., 2006). Regular physical activity helps patients maintain their mobility and muscle strength (Hochberg, et al., 1995a; Holman and Lorig, 1997; Managing Osteoarthritis, 3/14/2006). Walking, aquatics, or similar types of exercise improves aerobic capacity and stamina while at the same time reduces feelings of anxiety and depression (Hochberg, et al., 1995a; Hochberg, et al., 1995b; Managing Osteoarthritis, 3/14/2006). It is critical that OA patients not attribute pain to the progression of OA because they may avoid exercise and physical activity. Instead, patients should attribute pain to the loss of muscle tone and strength since they may increase their participation in exercise to reduce this pain (Holman and Lorig, 1997; Managing Osteoarthritis, 3/14/2006).

Self-management programs may be beneficial for FM patients. Self-management programs offer training in coping skills such as relaxation techniques, activity pacing, and problem-solving approaches and/or training in physical exercise such as cardiovascular fitness, strength, and endurance training (Sandstrom and Keefe, 1998).

Despite the patient education and self-management efforts, physical activity levels among arthritis sufferers have been found to be sub-optimal. Using the 2002 National Health Interview Survey, Shih, et al. (2006) showed that 37% of adults with arthritis were not physically active, and adults with arthritis had a lower probability than adults without the condition of participating in recommended moderate or vigorous physical activity. Several risk factors were related to being physically inactive in both women and men with the condition: older age, low educational attainment, and functional disabilities. The researchers identified additional risk factors associated with physical inactivity in women: being Hispanic, being Non-Hispanic black, frequently suffering from anxiety and depression, having social impairments, requiring special equipment, and not obtaining counseling about physical activity. Among men, another risk factor related to physical activity was severe joint pain.

The investigators recommended helping arthritis sufferers gain better access to evidence-based interventions and physical activity programs. In addition, adults with arthritis should receive counseling about the importance of physical activity and pain management regimens that increase their participation in moderate and vigorous physical activity.

Another study found similar risk factors related to lack of recent exercise or physical activity among adults with arthritis (Fontaine and Haaz, 2006). Based on the 2004 Behavioral Risk Factor Surveillance Survey, Fontaine and Haaz (2006) found that older age, being African-American, and joint-related impairments were associated with not participating in recent exercise or physical activity. Other factors associated with lack of recent exercise or physical activity were being overweight or obese and reporting poor health. These researchers recommended addressing barriers to physical activity in arthritis sufferers and targeting sub-groups who are sedentary.

8
Cardiovascular Disease in the Elderly

Complications

As people age, they are at increased risk for developing cardio-vascular disease. The most prevalent sub-type of hypertension in the U.S. population is isolated systolic hypertension, once viewed as part of the normal aging process, is usually the result of increasing vascular calcification, or stiffening disease (Franklin, 2006). Stiffening disease refers to an age-associated deterioration of the elastic elements of the thoracic aorta and is related to a widening of brachial pulse pressure, which in turn, is associated with an increased risk of negative cardiovascular outcomes. Diabetes mellitus (DM), renal dysfunction, and untreated or poorly controlled hypertension may also produce premature arterial stiffening disease, resulting in stiffening and hypertrophy of the left ventricle. People with these conditions are at risk for developing coronary heart disease (CHD), heart failure (HF), stroke, vascular dementia, and chronic kidney disease.

Based on data from 3,035 subjects in the Health, Aging, and Body Composition study, Butler, et al. (2006) evaluated the metabolic syndrome and the risk of cardiovascular events in adults, aged 70 to 79 years of age. The metabolic syndrome is a cluster of risk factors which include, impaired glucose regulation, insulin resistance, raised arterial pressure, increased plasma triglycerides, and central obesity. The investigators found that patients with the metabolic syndrome had a greater risk of having coronary events, a myocardial infarction (MI), and a HF-related hospital stay than those without this syndrome. Women and whites with the metabolic syndrome had a higher rate of coronary mortality than those without this syndrome. Diabetic patients with the metabolic syndrome also had a higher rate of coronary events than those without this syndrome. The investigators conclude that patients over

70 years have a high risk for cardiovascular events, and the metabolic syndrome in this group is related to a greater risk of cardiovascular events.

Older individuals have a greater risk of dying after a heart attack and having complications than younger individuals (http://www.merck.com/mmhe/print/sec03/ch033/ch033c.html). One factor that may exacerbate these outcomes is that older individuals may suffer unusual symptoms, such as breathlessness, gastrointestinal complaints, stroke and/or disorientation. However, two thirds of older people report the usual chest pain, but they take longer than younger persons to admit that they are sick or to obtain emergency medical care.

Socioeconomic status (SES) and institutionalization factors can influence the extent to which this population may develop cardiovascular complications. Some patients lack the money to purchase the medications necessary to follow their medical regimen to and thus avoid complications. Others with little education, or with cognitive impairments may be unable to follow the doctor's orders. In a study of risk factors for early emergency hospital readmission in Hong Kong, Chu and Pei (1999) studied 380 patients aged 65 years or over and 380 matched controls, and found that having congestive heart failure (CHF) and no income were related to early emergency readmissions.

Demographic factors such as age, marital status, and gender may be related to risks for complications. Berkman, et al. (1991), in his investigation of 628 cardiac patients, found that older persons and those who had difficulty coping had a higher probability of being readmitted.

Some studies have found that women seem to have increased short-term and long-term mortality after an acute myocardial infarction (AMI) than men (Jiang, et al., 2006). Based on samples of 1,246 men and 537 women with AMI, Jiang, et al. (2006) discovered that women had a higher in-hospital mortality rate than men. Compared with men, women were older, had a higher rate of hypertension, DM, hyperlipidemia, and a higher Killp class of cardiac function. In addition, women were less likely to use reperfusion therapy and beta-receptor blockers compared to men. The authors suggest that these factors may explain why women had a higher in-hospital mortality rate than did men.

Based on a sample of 2,741 patients presenting with acute ST elevation myocardial infarction (STEMI), Cohen, et al. (2005)

showed that female gender was not an independent predictor of not receiving reperfusion therapy. Among women, older age and delayed presentation predicted not receiving reperfusion treatment and poorer outcomes. The authors recommend increased awareness especially among women to reduce delayed presentation after symptom onset.

Heer, et al. (2002) evaluated 6,067 consecutive patients with STEMI and found that there was a trend toward a higher in-hospital mortality rate in women. However, there were no gender differences in long-term mortality rates. Compared to men, women were 9 years older, had a higher rate of hypertension, DM, recurrent angina, and congestive HF. Women were less likely to have a history of a previous MI. Women had a longer pre-hospital delay, a higher rate of anterior wall infarction and were less likely to receive reperfusion than men.

A prospective study of 4,255 consecutive women 8,076 men who developed AMI in 19 hospitals in Seattle, Washington, also showed that women had a higher in-hospital mortality rate, but survival after hospital discharge did not vary based on gender (Maynard, et al., 1997).

Investigations also have found a significant interaction between gender and age in patients treated for AMI (Berger and Brown, 2006). These studies have shown that after being medically treated for AMI, younger women have a higher mortality rate than younger men, but the mortality rates for older women and men do not differ significantly. Berger and Brown (2006) evaluated possible gender-age interaction in 9,015 consecutive patients who received a primary angioplasty for AMI. They discovered that among patients under 75 years of age, women had a 37% increased risk of in-hospital mortality, while in patients 75 years and older, there were no gender differences in in-hospital mortality. The authors conclude that female gender is an independent predictor of in-hospital mortality in patients under 75 after receiving a primary angioplasty for AMI.

Roughly 20% of heart attack victims have only mild symptoms or no symptoms at all. This silent heart attack may only be recognized during a later physical exam when the physician does a cardiogram.

Many of those who survive a heart attack face life-threatening complications. Atrial fibrillation (AF) is a common complication of AMI and may increase the risk of mortality. Rathore, et al. (2000)

assessed AMI complicated by AF in a sample of 106, 780 Medicare beneficiaries, aged 65 years and older, from the Cooperative Cardiovascular Project. The researchers compared AF patients with non-AF patients to determine the prevalence and prognosis of MI complicated by AF. They discovered that 23,565 of the patients had documented AF, 11,510 had AF when presenting at the beginning of the hospitalization, and 12,055 acquired the condition during hospitalization. Compared to non-AF patients, AF patients were older, suffered more advanced heart failure, and were more likely to have suffered a previous heart attack and had a coronary revascularization procedure. The findings also revealed that AF patients had worse outcomes than non-AF patients. Relative to non-AF patients, those with AF had a higher mortality rate during hospitalization, a higher 30-day mortality rate, and a higher 1-year mortality rate. Patients who acquired AF during hospitalization had a worse prognosis than those who had the condition at the beginning of hospitalization.

More than 75% of CHF patients are over the age of 75 and this disease is a leading cause of hospitalization in older persons (Rich, 1997). In this population, at least 20% of hospitalizations are a result of heart failure (http://www.healthcentral.com/heart-disease/surviving-heartattack-000013_5-145_pf.html). Heart failure is the leading cause of death for persons over age 65 years. The basic pathophysiology of CHF is similar for both older and younger patients (Rich, 1997). However, older adults are more likely to develop diastolic HF, which consists of CHF combined with preserved left ventricular systolic function. This condition is present in up to 50% of all persons older than age 65 years with CHF.

Older adults suffering from a heart attack and HF are at increased risk for developing depression and cognitive impairment (Koenig, 2006; Qiu, 2006). Research has been underway to determine if older depressed hospitalized patients with CHF and/or chronic pulmonary disease differ from depressed patients with other medical problems. Koenig (2006) compared depressed hospitalized patients having CHF/chronic pulmonary disease with depressed patients who had other medical conditions. The results showed that among patients with major depression, those with CHF and/or chronic pulmonary disease had less severe symptoms of depression and cognitive dysfunction and more severe medical problems than depressed patients with other medical conditions. Among depressed hospitalized patients with minor depression, patients with CHF/chronic pulmonary disease were more likely to be older. Like those with major depression, patients with minor depression tended to have less severe depression and more serious medical problems.

Although research has found an association between HF and cognitive dysfunction in aged individuals, little is known about the possible link between heart failure and the risk of dementia. Using a population-based cohort study of 1,301 persons aged 75 years and older, Qiu, et al. (2006) evaluated the risk of persons developing dementia and Alzheimer disease (AD) over a 9-year period. Their findings indicated that 440 persons were diagnosed with dementia, including 333 with AD based on 6,534 person-years of follow-up. HF was found in 205 of the participants at the beginning of the study. HF was related to an increased risk of dementia and AD. Moreover, HF combined with low diastolic pressure added to the risk of developing dementia.

Disability and Quality of Life

Elderly individuals who have suffered cardiovascular events can suffer from significant disability and quality of life losses, which in turn can result in a variety of physical, cognitive, and psychosocial impairments.

Ades, et al. (2002) studied the relative role of medical factors, gender, fitness, and psychosocial conditions in predicting physical functioning in coronary patients older than 65 years. Their results indicated that peak aerobic capacity and depression were the conditions that best predicted physical functioning. The findings also revealed that women had worse physical functioning than men even though they had similar age, diagnosis, depressive symptoms and co-morbid health problems.

Using data from 265 post-MI patients in the Cardiac Rehabilitation in Advanced study, Marchionni, et al. (2000) analyzed the determinants of exercise tolerance following AMI in older patients. According to their results, older age, female gender, a small body surface area, a low amount of physical activity prior to the MI, and post-MI depressive symptoms predicted lower exercise tolerance. Increasing age is associated with 70% of the decrease in exercise tolerance. However, physical activity and depression, which are modifiable conditions, also should be included in the assessment and treatment of elder post-MI patients.

In Italy, Boccia, et al. (2005) studied age- and gender-associated use of cardiac procedures and interventions based on a retrospective analysis of 2,805 patients in six regions. Their results showed that patients over 75 years of age were less likely to receive a percutaneous transluminal coronary angioplasty and thrombolysis than younger patients. In contrast, aged patients were more likely to receive a permanent pacemaker than younger patients. No gender differences were found in the use of cardiac techniques.

Based on a study of 1,298 patients hospitalized with acute worsening of CHF, Auerbach, et al. (2000) found that African-Americans who had incomes less than $11,000 or who were over 80 years of age had a lower chance of receiving care from a cardiologist. However, patients with a college education were more likely to receive cardiologist care.

Medicaid status is also a determinant for the receipt of proper diagnostic and treatment procedures. Philbin, et al. (2001) analyzed the use of cardiac procedures among Medicaid patients based on a study of 11,579 patients hospitalized for acute MI. They discovered that Medicaid patients were less likely to have a cardiac catheterization, percutaneous transluminal coronary angioplasty and any type of revascularization technique.

Being married has been found to be associated with decreased physical impairment in individuals with hypertension and may predict less functional disability in older heart disease patients. Morewitz (2004), based on data from the National Health Interview Survey, found that married individuals living with their spouses were less likely to report that hypertension impaired their activities than non-married individuals.

Psychosocial conditions such as anxiety and depression are major predictors of increased disability, morbidity, and mortality in aged cardiac patients. Using a sample of 284 patients, aged 65 and older, hospitalized with an AMI, Romanelli, et al. (2002) found, that when compared with non-depressed individuals, those with depression had a greater chance of dying four months after discharge from the hospital, and that they were less likely to follow a physician's recommended diet, i.e., a low-fat and low-cholesterol diet or a diabetic diet, than those without depression. Moreover, these patients had a lower probability of exercising regularly, dealing with stress appropriately and improving their social support than non-depressed patients.

Based on a cross-sectional study of 1,024 adults with stable coronary artery disease (CAD), Ruo, et al. (2003) analyzed the relative impact of psychosocial and physiological conditions on functional disability and health-related quality of life. They discovered that depressive symptoms predicted higher symptom burden, more physical disability, and lower overall health. In contrast, two standard measures of cardiac function, left ejection fraction and ischemia did not predict health-relate quality of life. Only one measure of cardiac function, reduced exercise capacity, was linked to decreased overall health status.

Most research on functional status and quality of life in HF patients has focused on patients in clinical trials (Gott, et al., 2006). These clinical trials frequently have excluded older individuals, women, and people with co-morbid health problems. Little is known about the disability level and quality of life of older persons with HF who are recruited from primary care settings.

Based on a sample of 542 persons, older than 60 years of age, in general practice surgery settings in the United Kingdom, Gott, et al. (2006) studied predictors of impairment and quality of life in older individuals with HF. Their findings indicated that older HF patients have reduced quality of life, especially for women, those with significant impairment, and those suffering from depression, and those who have two or more co-morbid health problems.

Few studies have compared older and younger HF patients in terms of their physical disability and health-related quality of life. Masoudi, et al. (2004) compared the functional status and health-related quality of life of 194 heart failure patients older than 65 years and 290 younger HF patients. They found that older HF patients had relatively good health-related quality of life despite major physical impairments. However, older HF patients who experienced increased functional disability during the study period suffered significant reductions in their health-related quality of life. The authors conclude that their study emphasizes the importance of preserving functioning in older HF patients, including those who have major baseline impairments.

Stress, Coping, and Social Support

Aged heart disease patients may develop anxiety, depression, cognitive impairment, low self-esteem, functional impairment, and become overly dependent on their caregivers and others. These problems can lead to significant risks for morbidity and mortality by limiting their ability to respond to the stresses of life threatening cardiac events. (Koenig, 2006; Romanelli, et al., 2002; Riegel and Dracup, 1992). They may lack the cognitive capacity to respond to novel, unexpected, and unpredictable situations such as trying to recover from an acute cardiac event (Sotile and Miller, 1998). Further institutionalization may increase their risk of cognitive and functional impairment.

Having feelings of mastery over the environment, self-efficacy, and having positive self-esteem are important psychosocial resources for coping with cardiovascular disease and reducing the traumatic effects of anxiety and depression (Penninx, et al., 1998).

Ai, et al. (2006), using 481 older patients undergoing cardiac surgery, discovered that patients who used religious coping techniques before surgery were more likely to have improved short-term global functioning after surgery. In a previous survey, in 2005, using data collected from 224 middle-aged and older patients one day before major cardiac surgery, Ai, et al. (2005) found that the use of private prayer predicted greater internal control. The authors referred to this coping strategy as an event-specific vicarious control technique.

In addition, socioeconomic status factors such as poverty can have substantial adverse effects on their functioning and ability to cope with their disease (Sotile and Miller, 1998).

Gender differences in coping have been found in patients who have suffered a MI, and these differences may also occur in aged heart disease patients (Kristofferson, et al., 2003). In a review of the literature, Kristofferson, et al. (2003) found that women who have a MI reported less social support than men, possibly because they often de-emphasized their physical discomfort and delayed going for treatment because they did not want to bother their caretakers/family. Studies have shown that some women who had a MI report that performing household tasks helped them recover from their disabilities, and men reported that returning to work and keeping physically fit was important to them. Compared to men, women received less information about their condition and cardiac rehabilitation.

Marital status may help to predict patients' ability to cope with their disease (Morewitz, 2004; Berkman, et al., 1991). In a study of risk factors for hospital readmission, Berkman, et al. (1991) found that fewer married patients were being readmitted than singles.

Marriage seems to provide the necessary social support that enhances the patients' sense of control that in turn helps them deal with their disease. Without this social support, they may develop a passive, learned helplessness that will interfere with cardiac rehabilitation by reducing the patient's ability to follow a medical regime (Sotile and Miller, 1988).

Social support for older cardiac patients can come in different forms, including emotional, financial support, etc. Penninx, et al. (1998) showed that emotional support can having a buffer effect on depressive symptoms. Having a partner and/or many close relationships are significant coping strategies that help patients to deal with anxiety and depression (Penninx, et al., 1998).

Depression, itself is a negative factor in the receipt of social support. Romanelli, et al. (2002). Sotile and Miller (1998) suggest that having family problems has a negative impact on the patient's ability to function and cope. On the other hand, Riegel and Dracup (1992) discovered that patients who received excessive support had experienced more favorable outcomes one month after an AMI and experienced less anxiety, depression, anger, and confusion than patients who lacked such support. They also reported more vigor and more positive self-esteem. Four months after an AMI, patients with inadequate support were more dependent.

Schwarz and Elman (2003), who interviewed 128 HF patient caretakers, found that when caretaker's, themselves, suffered from stress and/or depression, their charges were at increased risk for hospital readmissions.

Meller (2001), used a sample of 107 caregivers in Israel, to compare the well-being of caregivers of patients hospitalized with complications from heart disease and other chronic diseases with the caregivers of patients hospitalized with dementia. The author found that both groups of caregivers have a significant risk of developing physical and mental health problems and of having reduced social activity and increasing financial problems. Micik and Borbasi (2002) recommend starting stress management programs for spouse caregivers in order to reduce their stress levels.

Treatment and Rehabilitation Outcomes

Outcomes from Diagnostic and Treatment Procedures

The diagnosis and treatment of heart disease in aged patients is complicated by co-morbid health problems which can both worsen ischemic heart disease and interfere with drug and interventional treatments (Kaski and Smith, 2000). In addition, these co-morbid conditions complicate the diagnosis and treatment of patients with HF and other cardiac conditions (Rich, 2005).

Based on a review of 3,494 cardiac catheterizations performed at 28 military medical centers, Jackson, et al. (2000) showed that the possibility for complications from cardiac catheterization was high for patients who: 1. were over 60 years of age; 2. had hypertension and/or peripheral vascular disease; 3. had a previous angioplasty. Dumont, et al. (2006) assessed predictors of vascular complications after cardiac catheterizations and percutaneous coronary interventions with femoral artery access using a sample of 11,119 patients. Their predictors were: 1. being older than 70 years and/or female; 2. having suffered renal failure; 3. having undergone a percutaneous procedure or having a venous sheath.

Based on a six-year follow-up of 193 elderly cardiac surgery patients, Speziale, et al. (2005) found that the New York Hospital Association functional classifications: 1. cardiopulmonary bypass and cross-clamping time; 2. use of urgent procedures and ischemic mitral valve techniques, were predictive of an increased risk of hospital death.

Patients can have a favorable quality of life despite the risk of complications with coronary interventions. For example, a study of 100 patients classified into three age groups (under 60 years, 60-70 years, and older than 70 years) evaluated their quality of life following percutaneous coronary interventions (Moore, et al., 2006). The authors found that health-related quality of life improved in all three age groups.

Age may have a negative impact on patients who undergo non-cardiac surgery. Polanczyk, et al. (2001) used a prospective cohort study of 4,315 patients, aged 50 years and older, to assess the effects of age on perioperative complications, length of hospital stay, and mortality among patients who underwent non-emergency, non-cardiac surgery. Their findings revealed that aged patients had higher rates of perioperative cardiac and non-cardiac complications and mortality and a longer length of stay than younger patients. However, mortality was low even in patients aged 80 years and older.

Modifying the way acute hospital care is provided may enhance activities of daily living and quality of life following cardiac surgery. In the previously mentioned study, Speziale, et al. (2005) assessed the impact of a multi-dimension intervention on survival, disability, quality of life, and other outcomes. The intervention consisted of a uniquely-developed environment for elderly patients, and an inter-disciplinary focus that involves health providers during and after hospitalization. The results showed that the multi-dimensional intervention produced a total survival rate of 89.7%. In addition, the percent of patients who did not need re-hospitalization was 69.8%, and the percent of patients who did not need repeat surgery was 99%. Patients also had improved physical and psychosocial functioning, quality of life, and overall satisfaction.

Silver et al. (2006) suggest that emergency department-based HF observation units can reduce morbidity, mortality of utilization of health care resources. These HF observation units assist patients with taking their oral agents, including angiotensin-converting enzyme inhibitors, beta-adrenergic receptor blockers, and diuretics. These units also facilitate the use of vasoactive agents, effective HF education, and follow-up.

Cardiac Rehabilitation (CR)

CR is an essential part of secondary prevention and is recommended for patients with various heart problems, such as following an AMI and revacularization. (Fattirolli, et al., 2005; Beswick, et al., 2005). It has been found to be a safe and effective method for reducing long-term morbidity and mortality and enhancing a variety of other out-comes, including strength, aerobic fitness, endurance, and physical functioning.

Despite the fact that a majority of cardiac hospitalizations and procedures are for elderly patients, many of those with severe dis-ease, may be less likely to be referred and/or less likely to par-ticipate in these CR programs compared to non-elderly patients (Beswick, et al., 2004; Beswick, et al., 2005; Paquet, et al., 2005). Based on an analysis of United Kingdom hospital discharge sta-tistics, Beswick, et al. (2004) discovered that not only did older individuals and women have low rates of referral and participa-tion in CR programs, but so did ethnic minority patients and patients with angina. Patients with angina or HF also had low rates of referral and attendance in CR.

Most studies of CR have emphasized younger patients, thus resulting in a paucity of research on older age groups (Fattirolli, et al., 2005; Ferrara, et al., 2006). Fattirolli, et al. (2005) suggest that

CR for the older patient should emphasize preserving mobility, independence and cognitive functioning. Therefore, research should focus on discovering more efficacious procedures for helping patients maintain their physical functioning and individual autonomy (Aggarwal and Ades, 2001).

Sinclair, et al. (2005) note that hospital- and exercised-based CR programs may not be as beneficial as home-based CR programs for many patients. Their study involved two groups of patients aged 65 or older, who had been discharged from the hospital following a suspected MI. One group received standard CR therapy, the second group received therapy at home, by a nurse, who visited them 1 to 2 weeks and then 6 to 8 weeks after their discharge. At these visits, the nurse provided education, emphasized adherence to the patient's regimen, encouraged the patient to resume daily activities, and gave appropriate referrals to community resources. Patients in the intervention group had fewer hospital readmissions and fewer days of hospitalization after initial discharge. At follow-up, 98% of the patients had resume driving, compared to 74% in the standard care group. There were no differences in activities of daily living, quality of life, and mortality rates between the two groups. However, patients in the intervention group had higher levels of self-confidence and self-esteem than those in the standard care group.

There is little evidence to determine if patients older than 75 years of age can benefit from CR since they have been excluded from most clinical trials (Marchionni, et al., 2003; Vigorito, et al., 2003). These individuals are more likely to suffer frequent co-morbid health problems, disability, psychosocial problems, cognitive impairment and high rates of morbidity and mortality. Therefore, it is necessary to ascertain which types of CR, if any, would be helpful for this population (Vigorito, et al., 2003; Marchionni, et al., 2003).

In Marchionni, et al. (2003)'s study, 270 patients after a MI were randomly selected into the following three groups: 1. an outpatient, hospital-based CR; 2. a home-based CR, 3. no CR. Each of the subgroups was classified into 3 age groups (45 to 65 years; 66 to 75 years; and over 75 years). The investigators showed that in each age group, total work capacity improved in the short term among patients in the hospital-based CR and the home-based CR programs but did not improve among patients in the control group. Patients in both the 45 to 65 and 66 to 75 year age groups had similar improvements in total work capacity. Short-term improvement was smaller in the over 75 age group, although still significant. Among patients in the hospital-based CR program, total work capacity deteriorated to the baseline level, while total work capacity did not revert to baseline level in the home-based CR group. The home-based CR had lower costs than the hospital-based CR. The investigators conclude that home-based CR may be the best choice for older patients because of the lower costs and more sustained positive outcomes.

Researchers are also investigating the impact of resistance training on aged patients with CHD and physical impairments. Resistance training is a type of strength training in which each effort is performed against a specific opposing force created by elastic resistance. Using a sample of disabled older women, Ades, et al. (2005) compared the effects of a progressive 6-month resistance training program with a control group whose therapy consisted of low-intensity yoga and deep breathing. Participants in the progressive 6-month resistance program had higher rates of physical activity energy and total energy expenditure than those in the control group. Those in the resistance program achieved significant increases in upper and lower body strength but had no change in fat-free mass or left ventricular function.

Patient Education and Self-Management

It is a given, that one's knowledge and understanding of one's own medical condition can foster the self-care practices and lifestyle modifications necessary to deal with that condition (Beswick, et al., 2004). Patients' self-care practices can involve taking prescribed medications, managing stress, exercising, monitoring weight, following recommended sodium restrictions, monitoring symptoms (Gary, 2006; Clark and Dodge, 1999).

According to Artinian, et al. (2002), some HF patients are especially deficient in their knowledge about medications, monitoring their weight, and recognizing the meaning and symptoms of HF. In their study of patients with chronic stable angina (mean age 63 years), Kimble and Kunik (2000) reported that 65% of the patients in the sample did not know how to use sublingual nitroglycerin to prevent symptoms. In addition, they found that 32.6% of the patients used sublingual nitroglycerin for symptoms not related to chest pain.

The complexity of the medical regimen can make it very difficult for patients to follow their regimens. The presence of co-morbid cardiac and non-cardiac problems may interfere with self-care practices. The high rates of cognitive impairment and depression in older populations make self-care practices even more problematic for patients suffering these problems.

Artininian, et al. (2002) showed that high levels of education predicted higher levels of knowledge about their disease among HF patients. It is highly likely that patients with little formal education may not understand the total ramifications of their disease and the importance of following medical personnel's orders. This group may also have limited financial resources and be unable to afford the necessary components of their prescribed medical regimens.

In Spain, Gonzalez, et al. (2004) used nurses' evaluation of 324 patients in a new multidisciplinary HF unit to show that older patients had a lower level of knowledge about certain aspects of their disease and were less physically active than younger patients.

In Gonzalez, et al. (2004)'s investigation, women had a lower level of knowledge about their condition and engaged in less physical activity than men. The authors also found that older patients and women actually did better in following their prescribed sodium restriction and had better smoking and drinking habits than younger patients and men. Artinian, et al. (2002) found that older age was related to higher levels of knowledge about their disease among HF patients.

The lack of social support and the high rates of hypertension impairment among non-married persons may reflect their difficulties in following self-care practices (Morewitz, 2004).

Research is underway to determine the impact of interventions on self-care practices in older cardiac patients (Gary, 2006; Gonzalez, et al., 2004). Emphasis has been on assessing the effects of interventions on self-care practices and health care utilization and costs. Investigators have analyzed the impact of patient education on improving psychosocial functioning and preventing disease complications. Researchers are also focusing on improving the role of clinicians in promoting self-care and other positive health care outcomes.

Lacey, et al. (2004) evaluated the impact of a self-help package, the Heart Manual using a controlled observational study design.

They compared two cohorts of patients following hospitalization for an AMI. One cohort received the Heart Manual in addition to standard care and the control cohort just received standard care. The findings revealed that participants in the intervention cohort did significantly better in reducing their feelings of anxiety and depression three months after hospitalization. Patients over age 80 and those who participated in hospital-based rehabilitation classes also showed improvements. The investigators conclude that the Heart Manual, combined with hospital-based rehabilitation education, are effective and patients of all ages can benefit from these interventions.

Using a sample of 179 patients (mean age of 73 years) hospitalized for HF, Jaarsma, et al. (1999) evaluated the impact of education and support compared to a control group who received the usual care. The intervention group received intensive training about the effects of HF on their activities from a study nurse. Patients received education and support during their hospitalization and during a home visit within one week of discharge. The findings revealed that those patients in the intervention group had higher rates of self care than the control group. However, the two groups did not differ in their use of health care services.

Wheeler, et al. (2003) assessed the impact of a heart disease self-management program on health care utilization and costs for older women (233 in the intervention and 219 in a control group) diagnosed with heart disease. The intervention consisted of the Women Take PRIDE program, which uses a self-regulation process for promoting older women's adherence to their medical regimen. The results of the study indicated that those in the intervention group had fewer in-patient days than those in the control group. Hospital cost savings produced by the intervention exceeded intervention costs by a ratio of almost 5 to 1. The authors conclude that a heart disease self-management intervention program can lower health care use and has the potential to reduce costs for health plans.

Clark, et al. (1992) investigated the effects of self-management training on the functional health status of 324 older individuals with cardiac disease. They randomly assigned the women and men to either a self-management education program or a control group. Their findings indicated that persons in the intervention program had higher psychosocial functioning and well-being than those in the control group.

A major concern is ensuring that health care providers have the knowledge, skills, and attitudes to effectively promote self-care practices in elder heart disease patients. Based on a retrospective medical record review of discharge instructions for HF patients, age 65 and older, Lesperance, et al. (2005) discovered that nurses were lax in teaching hospitalized patients about the importance of there was a lack of nursing attentiveness to teaching hospitalized patients about monitoring weight gain. Furthermore, there was no emphasis on making referrals to patients when they were discharged from the hospital.

Dykes, et al. (2005) assessed the impact of improving clinicians' adherence to clinical practice guidelines for HF patients. The authors evaluated health providers' adherence to clinical practice guidelines before and after the implementation of the Heart Failure Effectiveness & Leadership Team (HEARTFELT) intervention, compared to a control group. The HEARTFELT program involved the use of several tools: 1) an automated pathway in the electronic medical record that contained medical orders, an interdisciplinary management plan, and self-care plan, 2) HF self-management education tools, 3) access to evidence for health care providers and patients, and 4) continuous, discipline-specific feedback about patient adherence. The findings of the study revealed that the intervention resulted in improvements in clinician adherence with self-management guidelines in the electronic medical record and clinicians' adherence with self-management education provided to patients at the time of hospital discharge. However, patients in the intervention and control groups did not differ in rates of adherence with medical regimen. The program worked as far as improving the medical record keeping, and the clinicians' adherence to standards, but it had no positive impact on patients. More research is needed to see what modifications need to be made so that patients' outcomes are more positive.

9
Seniors with Cancer

Approximately two-thirds of all solid tumors develop in individuals, aged 65 years and older (Audisio, et al., 2004). With the population aging, and the resulting increase in life expectancy, more people will develop cancers, such as breast, gastrointestinal tract, and lung cancers (Ramesh, et al., 2005). Therefore, it is surprising that few randomized controlled trials have been performed to test new cancer treatments in this population (Bernardi, et al., 2006; Audisio, et al., 2004; Repetto, et al., 2003).

Risk Factors and Complications

Aging may be viewed as a loss of stress tolerance, which results in: 1. a lowering of the functional reserve of organ systems; 2. increased prevalence of co-morbid health problems; 3. reduced socioeconomic status (SES); 4. impaired cognition; 5. increased prevalence of depression (Ramesh, et al., 2005; Balducci and Extermann, 2000).

The aging process is highly variable, and the reasons for this variability are not well known (Repetto, et al., 2003; Balducci, 2003). Given this variability, it is necessary for clinicians to conduct a comprehensive geriatric assessment (CGA) with each of his or her patients in order to detect the reversible factors that may inhibit effective cancer therapy (Balducci, 2003; Repetto, et al., 2003; Balducci and Extermann, 2000; Roche, et al., 1997). These factors include depression, cognitive impairment, malnutrition, anemia, limited SES resources, and difficulties in social support and care giving.

In addition, there are pharmacological risk factors associated with treating cancer in the older patient for they can face decreased renal excretion of drugs and increased vulnerability to neutropenia and related infection, mucositis, cardiotoxicity, peripheral neuropathy, and central neurotoxicity (Rossi, et al., 2005; Repetto, 2003; Balducci, 2003; Balducci and Extermann, 2000). In addition, the progressive decline in organ system function, such as decreased stem-cell reserves, reduced ability to repair damaged cells, loss of body protein, and the pharmacokinetics of various chemotherapy agents, can produce increased toxicity of chemotherapy agents (Repetto, 2003).

The development of anemia can be a serious side effect of the disease, or its treatment, and if the anemia is not treated, drug functioning can be altered, increasing the risk of toxicity (Repetto, 2003).

Co-morbid health problems, which are more prevalent in the aged, are additional risk factors among older cancer patients (Rossi, et al., 2005; Repetto, 2003). Co-morbid conditions also increase the risk of toxicity because the medications used to treat to treat these problems may interact negatively with chemotherapy agents.

Pain, which results from cancer, its treatment, or other co-morbid diseases is another major risk factor (Balducci, 2003; Colleau, Pain in the elderly with cancer, http://www.whocancer pain.wisc.edu/eng/13_2/pain.html).

Disability and Quality of Life

Because of the variability of the aging process, it can be difficult to manage cancer in elderly individuals. Ramesh, (2005) feels that clinicians face an ethical dilemma in deciding how aggressive they should be in treating cancer patients. They need to know if patients will be able to tolerate the stress of anti-neoplastic treatment, as well as to determine if the treatment is more effective than detrimental to the patient.

Balducci and Extermann, (2000) believe that a CGA can help clinicians better assess the patient's life expectancy, level of functioning, tolerance for the cancer treatments, and desired quality of life. When using the CGA, practitioners are able to identify at least three stages of aging. In the first stage, the patients are functionally independent without co-morbid health problems, and thus should be able to tolerate any standard cancer therapy with the possible exception of bone marrow transplants. Second stage individuals have some functional impairment with co-morbid health problems. In this case, the initial chemotherapy dose would be reduced, but subsequent doses would be increased. If this approach is not feasible, then some other type of pharmacological treatment would be called for. Third stage patients are frail, for they are dependent on outside help in one or more activities of daily living (ADL), have three or more co-morbid health problems, and have one or more geriatric syndromes, such as cognitive impairment. Individuals in this stage are generally considered candidates for palliative treatment. However, it is important to note that the definition of frailty is controversial and not everyone agrees with the above criteria for determining who is frail (Repetto, et al., 2003). Therefore, the CGA should include a comprehensive evaluation of the patient's functional status, co-morbidities, tolerance for the treatments, life expectancy, etc. to ensure that the patients receive optimal care.

Quality of life and measures of functional status are used by clinicians and researchers to assess which factors influence changes in quality of life, physical and psychosocial functioning, and life expectancy in aged cancer patients undergoing cancer treatments.

Some studies have shown that quality of life, disability, and survival varies by the site and type of cancer. For example, in lung cancer patients over 65 years old, surgical risk increases and life expectancy is limited (Jaklitsch, et al., 2003). In contrast, five-year survival in colorectal cancer patients after potentially curative surgery has increased from 50% to 67% (Matasar, et al., 2004).

Despite suffering chemotherapy toxicities, Chen, et al. (2003) showed that those who suffered severe chemotoxicity had an even greater reduction in physical functioning than those who did not experience severe chemotoxicity.

In a study of changes in physical functioning following initial cancer therapy, Given, et al. (2001) found that pain, fatigue, and insomnia had negative effects on functional status independent of the type of therapy or co-morbid health problems.

Other research focuses on differences in functioning in cancer patients who undergo treatment and those who do not receive treatment. Roche, et al. (1997) showed that patients who did not receive cancer therapy had higher rates of functional disability than those who did receive treatment.

In addition, investigators have used quality of life and disability measures to determine the efficacy of specific single-agent and combination chemotherapy regimens. For example, in patients with advanced non-small-cell lung cancer, the ELVIS investigation showed that single-agent chemotherapy was effective with regard to quality of life and rates of survival (Di Maio and Perrone, 2003). The MILES investigation demonstrated that combination chemotherapy was not more effective than single-agent chemotherapy. The MILES study also revealed that quality of life at the beginning of the study was strongly associated with the prognosis of these patients (Di Maio and Perrone, 2003).

Pain and its treatment in aged cancer patients can impair their quality of life (Colleau, Pain in the elderly with cancer, http:// www.whocancerpain.wisc.edu/eng/13_2/pain.html). However, the actual assessment of pain in these patients can be especially difficult for they frequently underreport their pain.

Various other psychosocial conditions, such as depression and anxiety, can influence quality of life, functional status, and life expectancy in older cancer patients (Mehnert, et al., 2006; Maly, et al., 2005; Pedro, 2001; Kurtz, et al., 2002). In a cross-cultural survey of German, Japanese, and South Korean patients, Mehnert, et al. (2006) showed that depression reduced health-related quality of life (HRQL) in breast cancer patients.

In a study of 211 lung cancer patients, aged 65 years and older, Kurtz, et al. (2002) found that decreased functioning and greater symptom severity predicted higher depression. In addition, the investigators discovered that those patients who had not obtained radiation therapy had higher levels of depression than those who had been treated before the study.

Reduced social functioning can be associated with severe psychosocial distress, including Post Traumatic Stress Disorder (PTSD) in this population. Kornblith, et al. (2003) evaluated the long-term adjustment of early-stage breast cancer survivors using data from 153 women who had previously participated in a phase III randomized trial. They showed that those who reported that lymphedema and numbness had disrupted their social functioning were more likely to have greater symptoms of PTSD than those who had fewer symptoms of lymphedema and numbness. Other factors such as more severe negative life events and more dissatisfaction with patient care also predicted more PTSD symptoms.

Level of self-esteem may be an important determinant of quality of life in aged cancer patients. Using a sample of 456 long-term cancer survivors, Pedro (2001) showed that higher levels of self-esteem predicted higher HRQL.

It is difficult to assess the quality of life, functional status, and health problems in cognitively impaired individuals, particularly in the area of pain evaluation. Since many of these patients become non-verbal when they are in pain, clinicians need to be aware of behavioral changes that indicate the presence of pain (Colleau, Pain in the elderly with cancer, http://www.whocancer pain.wisc.edu/eng/13_2/pain.html).

Demographic and SES factors may affect level of quality of life (Parker, et al., 2003; Lehto, et al., 2006; Ganz, et al., 2003). Ganz, et al. (2003) found that, after breast surgery, younger women had improvements in their physical and mental health, whereas older women showed deterioration in their physical and mental health status.

Stress, Coping, and Social Support

According to a pilot study by Houldin and Wasserbauer (1996), two thirds of aged cancer patients surveyed reported that they had concerns or problems related to their condition. Almost 50% of the patients noted, felt that they had received insufficient emotional support, and 69% percent indicated that their spiritual support was inadequate.

A variety of factors can affect older cancer patients' ability to cope effectively with their condition and meet their diverse psychosocial, physical, and informational needs. Disease severity and treatment status may be predictive of coping effectiveness (Kornblith, et al., 2003). Patients with severe symptoms seem to have greater difficulty in coping with their condition. In addition, those patients who have not been in treatment may have decreased coping effectiveness and associated decreased functioning and psychosocial well-being (Kurtz, et al., 2002). Ranchor, et al. (2002) evaluated pre-morbid predictors of psychosocial adjustment to cancer in older patients and found that high neuroticism predicted higher levels of distress. Similarly, Penninx, et al. (1998) showed that perceiving mastery over the environment, expecting self-efficacy, having a partner, enjoying close social ties plus high levels of self-esteem reduced depressive symptoms in this population.

Social support is diverse and may be most effective when the support provided is consistent with the support needs of the patient (Robinson and Turner, 2003).

In the previously mentioned study, Penninx, et al. (1998) found that such factors as having a partner and having numerous close social ties predicted fewer depressive symptoms in older patients with chronic diseases and those without these conditions.

Based on a cross-sectional survey of 222 newly diagnosed breast cancer patients, aged 55 years and older, Maly, et al. (2005) discovered that patients having supportive partners and well-adjusted partners and children had lower levels of depression and anxiety. Among racial/ethnic minorities, having supportive and well-adjusted adult children was especially important.

Chan, et al. (2004) evaluated social support and coping in Chinese patients undergoing cancer surgery. Based on a sample of 60 patients from two regional hospitals in Hong Kong, the authors found that following surgery, tangible and informational supports seem to be more effective than emotional support. In addition, more attention should be paid to older patients and those with lower educational attainment since they may have ineffective social support.

Researchers are looking into the problems of caregivers and family members involved with older cancer patients. Given and Sherwood (2006), in their review of the literature, conclude that positive caregiver interventions have the potential to reduce patients' re-admissions and interruptions of cancer treatment and to enhance the emotional well-being of both patients and their caregivers.

Treatment and Rehabilitation Outcomes

Breast Cancer

Two early investigations have demonstrated that older women were less frequently screened for breast cancer than younger women (Muss, 1996; Wanebo, et al., 1997). Based on state health department and tumor registry, Wanebo, et al. (1997) found that there was a lower rate of detection of pre-invasive cancer for women, aged 65 years and older, relative to those aged 40 to 49 years.

In the past, comprehensive breast cancer treatment and therapy for older women have been shown to be sub-optimal. In Wanebo, et al. (1997)'s study, women, aged 65 years and older with highly curable Stage IA and IB cancer, were more likely to receive limited surgery (26% only had lumpectomy) compared to 9.4% in younger patients. The investigators found that 5-year survival was much worse (63%) in patients treated with only lumpectomy than in those treated by mastectomy (80%) or lumpectomy with axillary dissection and radiotherapy (95%). Similar treatment outcomes were shown for patients with Stage II cancer.

A comprehensive assessment of the patient is essential. This assessment consists of a medical history, cancer staging, and an evaluation of the patient's health and environment which may interfere with treatment strategies (Boer, 2005). It is recommended that older women, including those older than 70 years and in fair to good health, should have a mammography yearly to every other year (Muss, 1996). Medicare will now pay for mammography every other year.

The few clinical trials that have been conducted with older women reveal that surgery, radiation, and chemotherapy are equally effective in older as well as younger women (Muss, 1996). Breast cancer surgery is safe for elderly women without co-morbid health problems and their operative mortality is low (Boer, 2005; Audisio, et al., 2004). Since body image is important for a majority of older women, they should be offered breast conserving surgical options, reconstruction, and adjuvant radiotherapy if the nodal staging allows them (Boer, 2005). The selective lymph sentinel node technique, which offers optimal nodal staging with low mor- bidity, should be used to select patients who are candidates for axillary dissection (Boer, 2005). Selective lymph sentinel is appro- priate for all patients with a tumor size less than three centimeters (depending also on the size of the mammary gland) and no clinical indicators of axillary involvement (Audisio, et al., 2004).

Older women should undergo axillary lymph node dissection level I to III, regardless of their age, if they have tumors larger than three centimeters with negative axilla or if they have any size tumor and positive axilla (Audisio, et al., 2004). Removing axillary lymph nodes is controversial even though axillary metastases can metasta- size as well and although chemotherapy is not helpful in always controlling axillary disease and recurrence rates after axillary dissection seem to be lower than after axillary irradiation.

Research has shown that older women do as well as their younger counterparts with radiation therapy, and older women tolerate radiation therapy well. Intraoperative radiation therapy seems to be a possible alternative to standard radiotherapy (Boer, 2005).

For frail women with early- to late- stage breast cancer, tamoxifen may be employed as beginning treatment (Muss, 1996). However, tamoxifen is not as effective as surgery for attaining local control on a long-term basis. For women who are high-risk, node-negative and for those who are node-positive regardless of receptor status, adjuvant tamoxifen should be contemplated. For high-risk, node-negative and node-positive women who are in good health and have life expectancy of more than five years, adjuvant chemotherapy should be undertaken.

Endocrine therapy is a standard therapy in older women in the adjuvant and metastatic setting since they are more likely to have well-differentiated tumors with estrogen and progesterone receptors (Boer, 2005; Muss, 1996). After all hormonal treatments have been tried, chemotherapy should be used for those with progressive disease. Since older women frequently take several drugs at the same time, this polypharmacy may result in clinical changes in cytoxic agent pharmacology (Boer, 2005). Supportive care should be undertaken to enhance patient compliance with chemotherapy. A variety of patients should do well on oral and weekly applied cytoxic therapies. Those who have been performing poorly may especially benefit from these treatments.

Colorectal Cancer

Studies have found that there is an increased prevalence of colorectal cancer in older age groups. Based on a sample of 8,077 patients with newly diagnosed colorectal cancer, Tekkis, et al. (2002a & 2002b) discovered that 30.7% of the cases were in the 65-74 years age group, 29.9% in the 75-84 years age group, and 9.3% in the age group 85 years and older.

Heriot, et al. (2006) found that age, along with a higher American Society of Anesthesiology grade, operative emergency, and metastases were independent predictors of postoperative mortality. Other studies, however have found that age is not predictive of postoperative mortality in colorectal cancer patients. One study by Latkauskas, et al. (2005), using a sample of colorectal cancer patients younger than 75 years (N = 532) and 75 years and older (N=154), revealed that age was not an independent risk factor for postoperative mortality. However, this investigation found that the older age group had lower rates of overall 5-year survival and cancer-associated 5-year survival than the younger age group.

Similarly, Bufalari, et al. (2006), using a sample of 177 rectal cancer patients, discovered that the rates of postoperative mortality in patients, aged 65 years and older were comparable to patients younger than 65 years. However, the older patients had worse overall survival, cancer-related survival, and disease-free survival than younger patients.

Latkauskas, et al. (2005) showed that preoperative complications and co-morbid health problems, more advanced disease, and higher rates of postoperative non-surgical complications predicted worse postoperative complications in aged colorectal cancer patients. Similarly, the Colorectal Cancer Collaborative Group (2000) note that aged patients have a higher rate of co-morbidity, enter the health care system with advanced disease, and are more likely to undergo emergency surgery. Up to 40% of elderly colorectal cancer patients are still treated for surgical emergencies, e.g., obstruction and or perforation (Audisio, et al., 2004; Koperna, et al., 1997; Ficorella, et al., 1999). These patients are more likely to receive palliative operations and less likely to receive preoperative neoadjuvant treatments and postoperative adjuvant therapies than younger patients (Koperna, et al., 1997; Ficorella, et al., 1999).

There have been dramatic improvements in colorectal cancer treatment in the last decades. More aged patients are being cured or those not curable are having their quality of life improved by innovations in surgery, radiotherapy, and chemotherapy (Matasar, et al., 2004). Although treatment for the elderly has not kept up with therapy for younger patients, clinicians are beginning to take aggressive approach and use multi-modal treatments for older patients.

Surgeons are now operating on aged colorectal cancer patients with greater frequency than in the past (Matasar, et al., 2004). Patients undergoing surgery also are having less postoperative mortality and more successful outcomes. Five-year survival has increased from 50% to 67% for patients undergoing curative surgery.

Aged patients may be able to benefit from advancements in surgical procedures. For example, total mesorectal excision (TME), which significantly reduces local recurrences, has resulted in significant improvements in rectal cancer (Kapiteijn and van de

Velde, 2002). Research has demonstrated that older patients who undergo low anterior resection and TME do no worse than younger patients who have the same procedures (Ho, et al., 2003; Audisio, et al., 2004).

A minimally invasive surgery, the laparoscopic-assisted colectomy (LAC) has become a viable alternative for patients with colon diseases. Some older patients have had the LAC, but more research is needed to establish the safety and effectiveness of this procedure and whether it is a real alternative to open colectomy (Patankar, et al., 2003). Thus far, only minimal and short-term advantages in quality of life outcomes have been found for LAC over open colectomy.

In selected patients, an alternative to formal resection is transanal excision of low rectal cancer (Gonzalez, et al., 2003). For tumors from the upper rectum, transanal endoscopic microsurgery (TEMS) is used. For curative resections, selection criteria include early T-stage, good or moderate differentiation, small tumor size, and negative miscroscopic margins (Gonzalez, et al., 2003). Patients who undergo TEMS have similar rates of recurrence and survival as those who get TME for early rectal cancer (de Graaf, et al., 2002; Audisio, et al., 2004).

Audisio, et al. (2004) suggest that emergency and semi-emergency endoscoping stenting should be regarded as alternatives for treating colorectal cancer emergencies. However, for aged patients with co-morbid health problems, the mortality and costs of these procedures are uncertain (Boorman, et al., 1999; Audisio, et al., 2004).

More patients are enrolling in clinical trials involving adjunctive treatment, and this has resulted in additional knowledge about the impact of single-agent and combined chemotherapy on aged patients (Matasar, et al., 2004). Clinical trials provide clinicians with information about the advantages and toxicities of various chemotherapy agents.

Patients who receive the standard adjuvant chemotherapy, fluorouracil-based treatments, tend to do better than those who do not receive these treatments (Matasar, et al., 2004; Honecker, et al., 2003). For patients with metastatic disease, systemic chemotherapy has produced longer survival, controlled symptoms, and improved quality of life (Honecker, et al., 2003). Research has shown that 71% of patients getting fluorouracil-based treatments have a 5-year survival compared to a 64% for those who do not get these adjuvant chemotherapy treatments (Matasar, et al., 2004). These treatments have been recommended for fit elderly patients who can tolerate cytotoxic therapy (Honecker, et al., 2003).

Studies have evaluated the effects of using irinotecan combined with fluorouracil-based treatments in older patients (Matasar, et al., 2004). This approach has produced a survival of two months longer than fluorouracil by itself. Researchers are also focusing on capecitabine, oxaliplatin, raltitrexed, and tegafur/uracil (UFT) in the treatment of older patients. Oxaliplatin and irinotecan have produced significant activity in treating patients with metastatic disease (Honecker, et al., 2003). However, their benefits have not been proven for older patients (Matasar, et al., 2004).

Lung Cancer

Lung cancer treatment for older patients has lagged behind treatment for younger patients. Age discrimination and prejudice toward the aged, belief in the ineffectiveness of treatment for this elderly patients and limited societal and financial resources are some of the obstacles to improving care for this population (Langer, 2002). Fewer surgical options have been offered to lung cancer patients, aged 65 years and older and elderly patients are treated less aggressively than younger patients (Audisio, et al., 2004; Dajzman, et al., 1996). Many practitioners avoid having surgery performed or minimize surgical procedures based on the age of the patient (Jaklitsch, et al., 2003; Dajczman, et al., 1996). It has been assumed that individuals in this age group are frailer, have less pulmonary reserve, are at higher risk for postoperative problems, and have lower active life expectancy than those in younger age groups (Audisio, et al., 2004). Audisio, et al. (2004) note that many of these expectations reflect age-based disparities in treatment, and there are little data to support these beliefs.

Recent innovations in evaluating the pre-operative risks of patients and surgical and anesthetic procedures have significantly reduced operative mortality and morbidity in older patients (Jaklitsch, et al., 2003). Therefore, lung cancer therapy for elder patients should not be denied based on the belief that surgery and other treatments are too dangerous. Instead, clinicians should perform a CGA to assess the risks for their older patients and develop optimal treatment strategies for this growing segment of the population (Gridelli, et al., 2005).

With regard to surgical options, thoracic surgery has been shown to be a safe and practical alternative for well-selected older patients (Audisio, et al., 2004). Thoracotomy and pulmonary resection have acceptable rates of operative mortality and should be considered since surgery provides the best possibility of a cure for patients with early-stage lung cancer.

Detection of lung cancer at an earlier stage should be emphasized since that would increase the number of patients who could benefit from minimal resections or video-assisted thoracoscopic resection (VATS) (Audisio, et al., 2004: Koizumi, et al., 2002). VATS is more beneficial than thoracotomy since it produces less blood loss, less injury to the chest wall, and minimal decline in vital capacity and other measures of post-operative performance (Audisio, et al., 2004). Research has demonstrated that there are no differences in long-term cancer-related survival between patients who undergo the VATS and those who undergo open surgery.

Performing wedge resections and other limited lung surgery also may reduce surgical complications in older patients when it is not possible to perform a lobectomy (Audisio, et al., 2004). For patients with non-small cell lung cancer, lobectomy is still the preferred procedure. However, wedge resections are an alternative for patients who have co-morbid health problems.

The first randomized trial of treatment for older patients with advanced non-small-cell lung cancer (NSCLC) demonstrated that single-agent vinorelbine was more effective for patients than supportive care by itself (Gridelli, et al., 2005). Patients who received single-agent vinorelbine had better survival and quality of life.

Fit aged patients with advanced NSCLC who are treated with platinum-based therapies perform as well or almost as well as patients younger than 70 years (Langer, 2002). However, aged patients frequently have a higher incidence of neutropenia and fatigue than younger patients. In the aged, platinum doses above 75 mg/m2 administered every 3 to 4 weeks are more toxic than are lower doses.

Based on a large randomized clinical trial, researchers found that gemcitabine in combination with vinorelbine were no more effective than either agent by itself (Gridelli, et al., 2005). After reviewing available evidence in the literature, Gridelli, et al. (2005) recommend that single-agent chemotherapy with a third-generation (vinorelbine, gemcitabine, a taxane) should be used for non-selected older patients with NSCLC.

Researchers have investigated the effectiveness of treatment for limited stage small-cell lung cancer (SCLC). Early meta-analysis revealed that chemo + radiation for SCLC patients older than 70 years of age was no more effective than chemotherapy by itself (Langer, 2002). In more recent studies, however, combined modality therapy has demonstrated an advantage for fit aged patients over those who receive chemotherapy alone.

Future research should evaluate the impact of co-morbid health problems on outcomes in elderly patients with lung cancer (Langer, 2002). Moreover, research on cancer patients over the age of 80 is warranted.

Prostate Cancer

Prostate cancer is the most prevalent non-skin cancer diagnosed in American men, and with the aging of the U.S. population, the management of prostate cancer is becoming a common problem for clinicians (Iowa Prostate Cancer Consensus Recommendations Committee; Dreicer, et al., 1996). Current guidelines focus on a starting age of the screening of prostate cancer but the age at which to discontinue screening has not been clearly delineated (Iowa Prostate Cancer Consensus Recommendations Committee). The effectiveness of prostate cancer screening is questionable, and indiscriminate use of prostate screening in aged men can lead to substantial costs and potential complications from procedures performed to evaluate abnormal screening test results or unnecessary treatment of prostate cancer (Volk, et al., 2003; Iowa Prostate Cancer Consensus Recommendations Committee). Therefore, it is necessary to have standard screening and management practices of prostate cancer in elderly men.

The Iowa Prostate Cancer Consensus Recommendations Committee has formulated recommendations for prostate cancer screening and management which use a risk-stratified approach (Iowa Prostate Cancer Consensus Recommendations Committee). These recommendations are designed to take into consideration the functional status and life expectancy of men aged 75 years and older.

According to these recommendations, prostate cancer screening for men, aged 75 years and older, with risk factors such as a positive family history and race (African-Americans) should only be started after a thorough discussion with the patients concerning treatment alternative and the benefits of treatment (Iowa Prostate Cancer Consensus Recommendations Committee). Men with a life expectancy of less than 10 years and with low grade/stage prostate cancer are not likely to get substantial survival benefit from treatment. Screening for prostate cancer should be done selectively if there is a high probability that the patient will not undergo treatment should cancer be diagnosed. If screening is undertaken, it is recommended that age-based prostate-specific antigen (PSA) screening values should be used to determine normal PSA levels.

In patients, aged 75 years and older, who have been previously screened, practitioners should have a thorough discussion of the risks and benefits of screening with these patients before continuing the prostate cancer screening (Iowa Prostate Cancer Consensus Recommendations Committee). These patients should realize that there is currently a lack of definitive knowledge that prostate cancer screening extends survival, especially in aged men. In men with a life expectancy of less than 10 years, co-morbid conditions, or who are not likely to adhere under go treatment, screening should be discontinued. However, in patients with symptoms indicative of prostate cancer, e.g., hematuria, bone pain, back pain, obstructive voiding problems, diagnostic PSA testing should be re-initiated.

Prostate cancer should be managed based on risk stratification, which predicts the probability of disease recurrence and prostate cancer-specific survival (Iowa Prostate Cancer Consensus Recommendations Committee). Patients with low or moderate risk of prostate cancer and a good chance of survival should be managed by watchful waiting and active surveillance. These patients should be treated once symptoms develop. Those patients at high risk for prostate cancer should receive radiation therapy with or without concomitant androgen ablation therapy. Assessment of the functional and cognitive status of the patient should be undertaken to assist in clinical decision making. Use of the Activities of Daily Living Scale, e.g., dressing, cleaning, and Instrumental Activities of Daily Living Scale, e.g., taking care of basic finances, are useful in determining functional status. Any impairment in basic or instrumental activities of daily living should trigger additional assessment before initiating treatment since their impairments may be indicative of co-existing health problems.

Taking into account the nature and severity of co-morbid health problems is very important in patients with prostate cancer. Patients in their eighties who have well or moderately differentiated localized prostate cancer with severe co-morbid conditions have a high probability of dying from causes other than prostate cancer (Wirth and Froehner, 2000).

Men who are diagnosed with prostate may be using complementary and alternative medicine, and this may affect their participation in conventional treatment. Using a population-based survey, Eng, et al. (2003) evaluated complementary and alternative medicine use in men recently diagnosed with prostate cancer.

Patient Education and Self-Management

More research is needed to determine the educational and self-management needs of aged cancer patients. One important question is whether older cancer patients differ in their information needs from their younger counterparts. Squiers, et al. (2005) analyzed 19,030 cancer patient calls made to the National Cancer Institute's Cancer Information Service between September, 2002, and August, 2003. They found that older cancer patients were more likely to inquire about specific treatment information than their younger counterparts. However, aged cancer patients were less likely to seek information about support services, psychosocial concerns, prevention activities, and risk factors.

A related area of research is older cancer patients' use of the Internet and its impact on their understanding of their condition and other outcomes. A prospective survey of 1,613 consecutive patients with cutaneous melanoma at the University of Michigan evaluated the prevalence and demographic correlates of Internet use that was related to their disease (Sabel, et al., 2005). The survey results indicated that younger patients were more likely to use the Internet to research their condition. The authors found 47% of patients less than 40 years of age conducted Internet research on melanoma, compared to only 12% of the patients aged 60 years or older. Neither gender nor disease severity was related to Internet use. About one third of those surveyed felt that the

Internet research reduced their anxiety, while a similar percentage believed that the Internet research increased their anxiety. Younger patients were more likely than older patients to report increased anxiety related to their Internet research on their condition. The authors suggest that clinicians become familiar with melanoma information on the Internet and assist their patients in using these online resources.

Other research has focused on health care disparities associated with the patient education and communication offered to aged cancer patients (Maly, et al., 2003; Maly, et al., 2006). Based on a sample of 222 older patients with newly diagnosed breast cancer, Maly, et al. (2003) evaluated factors associated with the extent to which physicians provide informational support to patients. Participants were asked about receiving and the helpfulness of 10 educational resources, such as booklets, videotapes and 15 examples of physician patient interactions, such as whether their physicians discussed the risk of disease recurrence and alternative treatments. Their findings showed that older age and Latina ethnic status were associated with less patient education and communication. Both older patients and ethnic minority patients indicated a preference for interpersonal sources over written sources of breast cancer information. However, both groups were less likely to receive interpersonal sources of information compared to younger patients. The authors suggest that enhancing the quality of clinician/patient communication and education may help to significantly reduce age and ethnic/racial disparities in the treatment of breast cancer patients.

Racial and ethnic differences in treatment decision-making and treatment received among elder cancer patients may be influenced by family preferences and level of acculturation. Maly, et al. (2006) discovered that about 49% of less assimilated Latinas and 18% of more assimilated Latinas reported that their family had made the decision about their treatment for breast cancer compared to less than 4% of African-Americans and whites.

Some researchers have explored the impact of clinician-patient communication on treatment outcomes, such as the selection of treatment and patient satisfaction among elderly cancer patients. Based on a sample of 613 pairs of surgeons and their patients, aged 67 years and older, who were diagnosed with localized breast cancer, Liang, et al. (2002) analyzed communication between physicians and patients and treatment outcomes. They showed that patients who reported being given various treatment alternatives were more likely to receive breast-conserving surgery with radiation than other types of therapy. Extensive physician-initiated communication was related to patients having the belief that they had a choice of treatment and satisfaction with their breast cancer care 3 to 6 months after surgery.

Maly, et al. (2004) revealed that surgeons who inquire about the treatment preferences of older breast cancer patients are more likely to have patients participate in their treatment. Moreover, the surgeons' solicitation of patient treatment preferences is associated with increased patient self-efficacy in communicating with their surgeons.

The training and practice characteristics of clinicians may also influence clinician-patient communication and treatment outcomes in aged cancer patients. In Liang, et al. (2002)'s investigation, surgeons who had been trained in surgical oncology were more likely to initiate communication with their breast cancer patients. Moreover, the authors found that surgeons who had a high-volume breast cancer practice had a higher probability of initiating communication with their breast cancer patients.

Various family, cultural, and health professional beliefs may create barriers to providing disease-associated information to older cancer patients (Brokalaki, et al., 2005; Hu, et al., 2002; Mitchell, 1998). Western medicine increasingly emphasizes full disclosure of cancer diagnosis or prognosis and the promotion of patient autonomy as essential aspects of ethical practice. However, families and physicians in some cultures are not truthful about a terminal diagnosis. Studies of European, Japanese, Native American, and different ethnic American cancer patients and physicians show that full disclosure of cancer is not preferred (Mitchell, 1998). Families and clinicians may believe it is better not to be truthful about the diagnosis and prognosis as a way of protecting that patient from the anxiety and trauma associated with a terminal diagnosis.

A Greek study of 203 hospitalized adult cancer patients evaluated demographic factors associated with awareness of diagnosis and medical information-seeking behavior (Brokalaki, et al., 2005). Using semi-structured, the investigators discovered that age was one of the factors that affected the patients' awareness of their diagnosis and their request for additional disease-related information. Older patients were less likely to be informed about their diagnosis and request more information than younger patients. With regard to other demographic factors, women and high school and university graduates had more knowledge about their diagnosis than men and elementary school graduates. Overall, over 50% of the patients interviewed reported that they were unaware of their diagnosis. The investigators conclude that the amount of information provided to patients is inadequate.

Based on a survey questionnaire of 250 palliative care workers at 15 Taiwan hospices, Hu, et al. (2002) analyzed possible family barriers to truthfulness in situations involving terminal cancer patients. They discovered several family-related barriers to truthfulness. First, some families did not know how to inform their older family member about a terminal cancer diagnosis and prognosis. Second, some families feel that it is not necessary to tell the truth to their aged family member. Third, there is a belief among families that aged family members can be happier without knowing about their terminal condition.

Mitchell (1998) suggests that clinicians should become aware of the cross-cultural differences in how people disclose issues related to cancer. They should be aware of the different preferences of patients. In addition, clinicians should be aware of the role of families in disclosing cancer information.

Without interventions, older cancer patients may have difficulty in performing self-care and self-management activities. Elder cancer patients are often faced with managing chemotherapy and radiation therapy side effects as well as the side effects and complications of cancer surgery. For example, older women with breast cancer often suffer the side effects of chemotherapy, including fatigue, anxiety, and sleep difficulty (Williams and Schreier, 2005).

Older breast cancer survivors often must manage the symptoms of lymphedema (Fu, 2005). Based on a qualitative investigation of women with breast cancer, Fu (2005) showed how some women can prevent lymphedema from worsening and are able to integrate the care of the disease into their daily activities.

In a study of radiation therapy for women with breast cancer, Wengstrom, et al. (2001) suggest that patients older than 50 years of age are especially at risk for having difficulties in coping with the demands of radiation treatment. Various age-related changes such as increased cognitive impairment, depression, and sleep difficulties are some of the factors that exacerbate aged persons ability to manage their treatment side effects. These conditions may reduce the person's self-efficacy in coping with the demands of cancer therapy and promoting healthy behaviors.

Based on a study of self-care among cancer patients, Lev, et al. (1999) reported that the patients' self-care self-efficacy decreased significantly over time. Similarly, the patients' quality of life and adjustment to cancer decreased substantially over time. They showed that decreased self-care self-efficacy was related to decreases in coping with cancer.

Researchers have analyzed various interventions designed to improve self-care and self-management behaviors among cancer patients. One investigation by Williams and Schreier (2005) evaluated the impact of educational audiotapes on breast cancer patients' self-care behaviors in managing the side effects of chemotherapy. Patients who received the educational audiotapes showed more self-care behaviors in managing chemotherapy side effects of fatigue, anxiety, and sleep problems. The authors discovered that patients who viewed the educational audiotapes engaged in more self-care behaviors, exhibited a wide range of these behaviors, and over time increased their use of these health promoting behaviors.

Based on a sample of 124 cancer patients, aged 21 years or older, at six urban cancer centers, Sherwood, et al. (2005) assessed the effectiveness of a cognitive behavioral intervention for patients with stage III, IV, or cancer recurrence. The cognitive behavioral program consisted of training patients in problem-solving techniques to reduce the severity of symptoms in an 8-week intervention that involved 5 contacts. The results indicated that symptom severity was reduced at 20 weeks, especially among patients aged 60 years and younger. The investigators suggest that cognitive behavioral programs can be effective in enhancing the problem-solving behaviors of advanced cancer patients, particularly those aged 60 years and younger.

Researchers have evaluated the impact of patient education on patients' participation in prostate cancer screening practices (Ruthman and Ferrans, 2004; Volk, et al., 2003). For example, Ruthman and Ferrans (2004) tested the efficacy of a video for teaching patients about prostate cancer screening and treatment. Based on a quasi-experimental design, they discovered that the video improved the participants' preference for PSA screening. However, the investigators showed that patients in the video intervention did not have more discussion with their physicians and their length of office visit did not increase.

Intervention programs are also being designed to increase cancer screening activities in older ethnic and racial populations. Women from ethnic and racial minority groups have especially low breast screening rates compared to white women, and this occurs in part because of financial difficulties (Kagay, et al., 2006; Fox, et al., 2001). To help overcome these financial constraints, Medicare in 1991 introduced subsidized biennial mammogram benefits. Fox, et al. (2001) analyzed the impact of targeted low-cost mailed intervention, informing women about the mammogram benefits. They discovered that among minority women who received the targeted mailed materials, mammogram use increased significantly. African-American women were two times as likely and Hispanic women were more than two times as likely to have mammograms compared to controls.

Racial and ethnic disparities in colorectal cancer incidence, mortality and use of colorectal cancer screening have been reported (Jandorf, et al., 2005). To help increase colorectal cancer screening among men and women, aged 50 years and older, in a minority community health setting, Jandorf, et al. (2005) tested the use of a patient navigator. They showed that patients who received patient navigator services were more likely to have a recommended endoscopic examination (15.8%) than those who did not receive the patient navigator services (5%).

In addition to financial factors, sociocultural factors may influence use of screening procedures in middle-age and elderly ethnic and racial minority populations (Yepes-Rios, et al., 2006; McCoy, et al., 1995). Knowledge about diseases, perceived health status, and having a discussion with a physician about screening procedures are factors that may affect screening rates in older minority populations.

References

About Arthritis, http://www.depuyorthopaedics.com

Adams, A.S., Mah, C., Soumerai, S.B., et al. (2003). Barriers to self-monitoring of blood glucose among adults with diabetes in an HMO: a cross sectional study. BMC Health Serv Res, 3 (1): 6.

Ades, P.A., Savage, P.D., Brochu, M., et al. (2005). Resistance raining increases total daily energy expenditure in disabled older women with coronary heart disease. J Appl Physiol, 98 (4): 1280-5.

Ades, P.A., Savage, P.D., Tischler, M.D., et al. (2002). Determinants of disability in older coronary patients. Am Heart J, 143 (11): 151-6.

Agency for Healthcare Research and Quality. (2002). Preventing disability in the elderly with chronic disease. Rockville, MD, Research in Action Issue 3. AHRQ Pub. No. 02-0018.

Aggarwal, A., Ades, P.A. (2001). Exercise rehabilitation of older patients with cardiovascular disease. Cardiol Clin, 19 (3): 525-36.

Ai, A.L., Peterson, C., Bolling, S.F., et al. (2006). Depression, faith-based coping, and short-term postoperative global functioning in adult and older patients undergoing cardiac surgery. J Psychosom Res, 60 (1): 21-8.

Ai, A.L., Peterson, C., Rodgers, W., et al. (2005). Effects of faith and secular factors on locus of control in middle-aged and older cardiac patients. Aging Ment Health, 9 (5): 470-81.

AirNow (2006). Older adults and air quality. http://airnow.gov/index.cfm.

Al Snih, S., Fisher, M.N., Raji, M.A., et al. (2005). Diabetes mellitus and incidence of lower body disability among older Mexican Americans. J Ger A Biol Sci Med Sci, 60 (9): 1152-6.

Albert Einstein Healthcare Network, Jefferson Health System. (2006). Common kidney problems, http://www.einstein.edu/yourhealth/kidney/article8550.html.

Aldwin, C.M. and Gilmer, D.F. (Eds.). (2004). Health, illness and optimal aging: Biological and psychosocial perspectives. Thousand Oaks, CA: Sage.

Aldwin, C.M., Levenson, M.R. and Gilmer, D.F. (2004). Interface between mental and physical health: An overview. Psychology and Health: Special Issue, Coping and Physical Health, 19, 277-282.

Allaire, S., Wolfe, F., Niu, J., et al. (2005). Work disability and its economic effect on 55-64-year-old adults with rheumatoid arthritis. Arthritis Rheum, 53 (4): 603-8.

American Cancer Society, Inc. (2006). Surveillance Research.

American Cancer Society, Inc. (2006). Press Room. 2006 World cancer declaration calls for global commitment to make cancer control top social and political priority.

American Geriatrics Society Foundation for Health in Aging. (2006).Back pain. http://www.healthinaging.org/agingintheknow/chapters_ch_trial.asp?ch=41.

American Geriatrics Society Foundation for Health in Aging. (2006). Managing the complications of diabetes in older persons. http://www.healthinaging.org/public_education/diabetes/managing_complications.php.

American Geriatrics Society Foundation for Health in Aging. (2006). Osteoporosis. http://www.healthinaging.org/agingintheknow/chapters_ch_trial.asp?ch=27.

Amoako, E.P., Richardson-Campbell, L., Kennedy-Malone, L. (2003). Self-medication with over-the-counter drugs among elderly adults. J Gerontol Nurs, 29 (8): 10-15.

Anderson, R.J., Freedland, K.E., Clouse, R.E., et al. (2001). The prevalence of comorbid depression in adults with diabetes: a meta-analysis. Diab Care, 24: 1069-78.

Andrew, T., Macgregor, A.J. (2004). Genes and osteoporosis. Curr Osteoporos Rep, 2 (3): 79-89.

Andrews, J.O., Heath, J., Graham-Garcia, J. (2004). Management of tobacco dependence in older adults: using evidence-based strategies. J Gerontol Nurs, 30 (12): 13-24.

Anstey, K.J. and Low, L.F. (2004). Normal cognitive changes in aging. Austral Fam Physician, 33, 783-787.

Anstey, K.J., Hofer, S.M. and Luszcz, M.A. (2003). Cross-sectional and longitudinal patterns of dedifferentiation in late-life cognitive and sensory function: the effects of age, ability, attrition, and occasion of measurement. J Exper Psych: General, 132, 470-487.

Araki, A. (2006). Diabetes education in elderly patients to maintain quality of life. Nippon Rinsho, 64 (1): 134-9.

Araki, A., Izumo, Y., Inoue, J., et al. (1995). Development of Elderly Diabetes Impact Scales (EDIS) in elderly patients with diabetes mellitus. Nippon Ronen Igakkai Zasshi, 32 (12): 786-96.

Arden, N., Nevitt, M.C. (2006). Osteoarthritis: epidemiology. Best Pract Res Clin Rheumatol, 20 (1): 3-25.

Armer, J., Fu, M.R. (2005). Age differences in post-breast cancer lymphedema signs and symptoms. Cancer Nurs, 28 (3): 200-7.

Armer, J.M., Heckathorn, P.W. (2005). Post-breast cancer lymphedema in aging women: self-management and implications for nursing. J Gerontol Nurs, 31 (5): 29-39.

Arnold, L.M., Hudson, J.I., Hess, E.V., et al. (2004). Family study of fibromyalgia. Arthritis Rheum, 50 (3): 944-52.

Aronow, W.S. (2006). Drug treatment of peripheral arterial disease in the elderly. Drugs Aging, 23 (1): 1-12.

Artinian, N.T., Magnan, M., Christian, W., et al. (2002). What do patients know about their heart failure? Appl Nurs Res, 15 (4): 200-8.

Audisio, R.A., Bozzetti, F., Gennari, R., et al. (2004). The surgical management of elderly cancer patients: recommendations of the SIOG surgical task force. Eur J of Cancer, (40): 926-938.

Auerbach, A.D., Hamel, M.B., Califf, R.M., et al. (2000). Patient characteristics associated with care by a cardiologist among adults hospitalized with severe congestive heart failure. SUPPORT Investigators. Study to Understand Prognoses and Preferences for Outcomes and Risks of Treatments. J Am Coll Cardiol, 36 (7): 2119-25.

Balducci, L. (2003). New paradigm for treating elderly patients with cancer: the comprehensive geriatric assessment and guidelines for supportive care. J Support Oncol, 1 (4 Suppl 2): 30-7.

Balducci, L., Carreca, I. (2002). The role of myelopoietic growth factors in managing cancer in the elderly. Drugs, 62 (Suppl 1): 47-63.

Balducci, L., Extermann, M. (2000). Management of cancer in the older person: a practical approach. Oncologist, 5 (3): 224-37.

Ballantyne, P.J. (2004). Social context and outcomes for the ageing breast cancer patient: considerations for clinical practitioners. J Clin Nurs, 13 (3a): 11-21.

Barnett, A., Birnbaum, H., Cremieux, P.Y., et al. (2000). The costs of cancer to a major employer in the United States: a case-control analysis. Am J Manag Care, 6 (11): 1243-51.

Barzilay, J.I., Spiekerman, C.F., Wahl, P.W., et al. (1999). Cardiovascular disease in older adults with glucose disorders: comparison of American Diabetes Association criteria for diabetes mellitus with WHO criteria. Lancet, 354 (9179): 622-5.

Barzilay, J.I., Kronmal, R.A., Gottdiener, J.S., et al. (2004a). The association of fasting glucose levels with congestive heart failure in diabetic adults > or = 65 years: the Cardiovascular Health Study. J Am Coll Cardiol, 43 (12): 2236-41.

Barzilay, J.I., Davis, B.R., Bettencourt, J., et al. (2004b). Cardiovascular outcomes using doxazosin vs. chlorthalidone for the treatment of hypertension in older adults with and without glucose disorders: a report from the ALLHAT study. J Clin Hypertens, 6 (3): 116-25.

Bastida, E., Cuellar, I., Villas, P. (2001). Prevalence of diabetes mellitus and related conditions in a south Texas Mexican American sample. J Comm Health Nurs, 18 (2): 75-84.

Bell, D.S. (1992). Exercise for patients with diabetes. Benefits, risks, precautions. Postgrad Med, 92 (11): 183-4, 187-90, 195-8.

Bell, R.A., Smith, S.L., Arcury, T.A., et al. (2005). Prevalence and correlates of depressive symptoms among rural older African Americans, Native Americans, and whites with diabetes. Diab Care, 28 (4): 823-9.

Berg, B. (1996). Aging, behavior and terminal decline. In J.E. Birren & K.W. Schaie (Eds.), The handbook of the psychology of aging (4th ed., pp. 323-327). San Diego: Academic Press.

Berger, J.S., Brown, D.L. (2006). Gender-age interaction in early mortality following primary angioplasty for acute myocardial infarction. Am J Cardiol, 98 (9): 1140-3.

Bergman-Evans, B. (2006). AIDES to improving medication adherence in older adults. Geriatr Nurs, 27 (3): 174-82.

Berkman, B., Millar, S., Holmes, W., et al. (1991). Predicting elderly cardiac patients at risk for readmission. Soc Work Hlth Care, 16 (1): 21-38.

Bernard, D.M., Banthin, J.S., Encinosa, W.E. (2006). Health care expenditure burdens among adults with diabetes in 2001. Med Care, 44 (3): 210-5.

Bernardi, D., Errante, D., Tirelli, U., et al. (2006). Insight into the treatment of cancer in older patients: Developments in the last decade. Cancer Treat Rev, 32 (4): 277-88.

Bertagnoli, R., Yue, J.J., Nanieva, R., et al. (2006). Lumbar total disc arthroplasty in patients older than 60 years of age: a prospective study of the ProDisc prosthesis with 2-year minimum follow-up period. J Neurosurg Spine, 4 (2): 8590.

Bertera, E.M. (2003). Psychosocial factors and ethnic disparities in diabetes diagnosis and treatment among older adults. Hlth Soc Work, 28 (1): 33-42.

Beswick, A.D., Rees, K., Griebsch, I., et al. (2004). Provision, uptake and cost of cardiac rehabilitation programmes: improving services to under-represented group. Health Technol Assess, 8 (41): iii-iv, ix-x, 1-152.

Beswick, A.D., Rees, K., West, R.R., et al. (2005). Improving uptake and adherence in cardiac rehabilitation: literature review. J Adv Nurs, 49 (5): 538-55.

Biessels, G.J., De Leeuw, F.E. Lindeboom, J., et al. (2006). Increased cortical atrophy in patients with Alzheimer's disease and type 2 diabetes mellitus. J Neurol Neurosurg Psychiatry, 77 (3): 304-7.

Birnbaum, H.G., Barton, M., Greenberg, P.E., et al. (2000). Direct and indirect costs of rheumatoid arthritis to an employer. J Occup Environ Med, 42 (6): 588-96.

Birren, J.E. (1974). Translations in gerontology: from lab to life: psychophysiology and speed of response. Amer Psychologist, 29, 808-815.

Birren, J.E. and Renner, V.J. (1977). Research on the psychology of aging: principles and experimentation. In J.E. Birren and K.W. Schaie (Eds.), Handbook of the psychology of aging. New York: Van Norstrand Reinhold.

Black, S.A. (1999). Increased health burden associated with comorbid depression in older diabetic Mexican Americans. Results from the Hispanic Established Population for the Epidemiologic Study of the Elderly survey. Diab Care, 22 (1): 56-64.

Black, S.A., Ray, L.A., Markides, K.S. (1999). The prevalence and health burden of self-reported diabetes in older Mexican Americans: findings from the Hispanic established populations for epidemiologic studies of the elderly. Am J Public Health, 89 (4): 546-52.

Blackman, L., Small, B.J. and Wahlin, A. (2001). Aging and memory: cognitive and biological perspectives. In J.E. Birren and K.W. Schaie (Eds.), Handbook of the psychology of aging. San Diego: Academic Press.

Blaum, C.S., Volpato, S., Cappola, A.R., et al. (2005). Diabetes, hyperglycaemia and mortality in disabled older women: The Women's Health and Ageing Study I. Diabet Med, 22 (5): 543-50.

Blazer, D.G. and Hybels, C.F. (2005). Origins of depression in later life. Psychol Med, 35 (9), 1241-1252.

Blazer, D.G., Hybels, C.F. and Pieper, C.F. (2001). The association of depression and mortality in elderly persons: A case for multiple, independent pathways. J Ger: Med Sci, 65A, M505-M509.

Boccia, A., Damiani, G., D'Errico, M.M., et al. (2005). Age- and sex-related utilization of cardiac procedures and interventions: a multicentric study in Italy. Int J Cardiol, 101 (2): 179-84.

Boer, K. (2005). Effective treatment strategy in elderly breast cancer patients. Orv Hetil, 146 (1): 15-21.

Bookwala, J., Harralson, T.L., Parmelee, P.A. (2003). Effects of pain on functioning and well-being in older adults with osteoarthritis of the knee. Psychol Aging, 18 (4): 844-50.

Boonen, A., van den Heuvel, R., van Tubergen, A., et al. (2005). Larger differences in cost of illness and wellbeing between patients with fibromyalgia, chronic low back pain, or ankylosing spondylitis. Ann Rheum Dis, 64 (3): 396-402.

Boonen, S., Autier, P., Barette, M., et al. (2004). Functional outcome and quality of life following hip fracture in elderly women: a prospective controlled study. Osteoporos Int, 15 (2): 87-94.

Boorman, P., Soonawalla, Z., Sathananthan, N., et al. (1999). Endoluminal stenting of obstructed colorectal tumors. Ann R Coll Surg Engl, 81, 251-254.

Bopp, K.L. and Verhaeghen, P. (2005). Explaining the many varieties of working memory variation: dual mechanisms of cognitive control. In R.A. Conway, C. Jarrold, M. Kane, A. Miyake and J. Towse (Eds.), Variation in working memory. New York: Oxford University Press.

Boyle, J.P., Honeycutt, A.A., Venkat Narayan, K.M., et al. (2001). Projection of diabetes burden through 2050. Diab Care, 24, 1936-1940.

Braun, A., Muller, U.A., Muller, R., et al. (2004). Structured treatment and teaching of patients with Type 2 diabetes mellitus and impaired cognitive function—the DICOF trial. Diabet Med, 21 (9): 999-1006.

Braver, T.S., Barch, D.M. and Keys, B. (2001). Context processing in older adults: evidence for a theory relating cognitive control to neurobiology in healthy aging. J Exper Psych: General, 130, 746-763.

Brenes, G.A., Guralnik, J.M., Williamson, J.D., et al. (2005). The influence of anxiety on the progression of disability. J Amer Ger Soc, 53 (1): 34-39.

Bressler, H.B., Keyes, W.J., Rochon, P.A. (1999). The prevalence of low back pain in the elderly. A systematic review of the literature. Spine, 24 (17): 1813-9.

Brokalaki, E.I., Sotiropoulos, G.C., Tsaras, K., et al. (2005). Awareness of diagnosis, and information-seeking behavior of hospitalized cancer patients in Greece. Support Care Cancer, 13 (11): 938-42.

Brown, A.F., Jiang, L., Fong, D.S., et al. (2005). Need for eye care among older adults with diabetes mellitus in fee-for-service and managed Medicare. Arch Ophthalmol, 123 (5): 669-75.

Brown, J.S., Seeley, D.G., Fong, J., et al. (1996). Urinary incontinence in older women. Who is at risk? Study of Osteoporotic Fractures Research Group. Obstet Gynecol, 87: 715-721.

Brown, S.C., Glass, J.M., Park, D.C. (2002). The relationship of pain and depression to cognitive function in rheumatoid arthritis patients. Pain, 96 (3): 279-84.

Brownie, S. (2006). Predictors of dietary and health supplement use in older Australians. Aust J Adv Nurs, 23 (3): 26-32.

Bruce, D.G., Davis, W.A., Cull, C.A., et al. (2003). Diabetes education and knowledge in patients with type 2 diabetes from the community: the Fremantle Diabetes Study. J Diab Complications, 17 (2): 82-9.

Bruce, D.G., Davis, W.A., Davis, T.M. (2005). Longitudinal predictors of reduced mobility and physical disability in patients with type 2 diabetes: the Fremantle Diabetes Study. Diab Care, 28 (10): 2441-7.

Bruckner, M., Mangan, M., Godin, S., et al. (1999). Project LEAP of New Jersey: lower extremity amputation in persons with type 2 diabetes. Am J Manag Care, 5 (5): 609-16.

Bruunsgaard, H. and Pedersen, B.K. (2000). Special feature for the Olympics: effects of exercise on the immune system: effects of exercise on the immune system in the elderly population. Immun Cell Bio, 78: 523-531.

Bucks, R.S. and Radford, S.A. (2004). Emotion processing in Alzheimer's disease. Aging and Mental Health, 8, 222-232.

Bufalari, A., Giustozzi, G., Burattini, M.F., et al. (2006). Rectal cancer surgery in the elderly: a multivariate analysis of outcome risk factors. J Surg Oncol, 93 (3): 173-80.

Bullock, K., McGraw, S.A. (2006). A community capacity-enhancement approach to breast and cervical cancer screening among older women of color. Health Soc Work, 31 (1): 16-25

Burge, R.T., Worley, D., King, A.B. (1997). Nationwide Inpatient Sample. Washington, D.C.: Agency for Healthcare Research and Quality.

Butler, J., Rodondi, N., Zhu, Y., et al. (2006). Metabolic syndrome and the risk of cardiovascular disease in older adults. J Am Coll Cardiol, 47 (8): 1595-602.

Butler, R.N., Forette, F. and Greengross, B.S. (2004). Maintaining cognitive health in an aging society. Journal of Research in Social Health, 124, 119-121.

Byrne, M.D. (1998). Taking a computational approach to aging: The SPAN theory of working memory. Psychology and Aging, 13, 309-322.

California Healthcare Foundation/American Geriatric Society Panel on Improving Care of Elders with Diabetes (2003). Guidelines for improving the care of the older person with diabetes mellitus. J Amer Ger Soc, 51 (10) Supplement: 5265-5280.

Calvo-Alen, J., Corrales, A., Sanchez-Andrada, S., et al. (2005). Outcome of late-onset rheumatoid arthritis. Clin Rheumatol, 24 (5): 485-9.

Caporali, R., Cimmino, M.A., Sarzi-Puttini, P., et al. (2005). Comorbid conditions in the AMICA study patients: effects on the quality of life and drug prescriptions by general practitioners and specialists. Semin Arthritis Rheum, 35 (1 Suppl 1): 31-7.

Carey, T.S., Evans, A.T., Hadler, N.M., et al. (1996). Acute severe low back pain. A population-based study of prevalence and care-seeking. Spine, 21 (3): 339-44.

Carney, C. (1998). Diabetes mellitus and major depressive disorder: an overview of prevalence, complications, and treatment. Depress Anxiety, 7: 149-57.

Caruso, L.B., Silliman, R.A., Demissie, S., et al. (2000). What can we do to improve physical function in older person with type 2 diabetes? J Gerontol A Biol Sci Med Sci, 55 (7): M372-7.

Caspi, A. and Roberts, B.W. (2001). Personality development across the life: the argument for change and continuity. Psychol Inquiry, 12, 49-66.

Castel, A.D. and Craik, F.I.M. (2003). The effects of aging and divided attention on memory for item and associative information. Psychology and Aging, 18, 873-885.

Center for the Advancement of Health (2005). Adalimumab Plus Methotrexate Effective for Long Standing Rheumatoid Arthritis. http://www.emaxhealth.com/97/3338.html.

Centers for Disease Control and Prevention (2002). Cancer-U.S. cancer statistics (USCS)-Facts and major findings-NPCR.

Centers for Disease Control and Prevention, Data and Trends, National Diabetes Surveillance System, Prevalence of diabetes, http://www.cdc.gov/diabetes/statistics

Centers for Disease Control and Prevention, National Center for Chronic Disease Prevention and Health Promotion. Chronic disease – press room. Atlanta, GA.

Centers for Disease Control and Prevention (2001). Diabetes and women's health across the life stages: A public health perspective. National Center for Chronic Disease Prevention and Health Promotion, Publications and Products, Fact Sheet, Atlanta, GA http://www.cdc.gov/diabetes/pubs/women/

Centers for Disease Control and Prevention (2005a). Lower extremity disease among persons aged > or = 40 years with and without diabetes—United States, 1999-2002. MMWR Morb Mortal Wkly Rep, 54 (45): 1158-60.

Centers for Disease Control and Prevention (2005b). Mobility limitation among persons aged > or = 40 years with and without diagnosed diabetes and lower extremity disease—United States, 1999-2002. MMWR Morb Mortal Wkly Rep, 54 (46): 1183-6.

Centers for Disease Control and Prevention (2005c). Prevalence of receiving multiple preventive-care services among adults with diabetes—United States, 2002-2004. MMWR Morb Mortal Wkly Rep, 54 (44): 1130-3.

Centers for Disease Control and Prevention (2004). Serious psychological distress among persons with diabetes—New York City, 2003. MMWR Morb Mortal Wkly Rep, 53 (46): 1089-92.

Centers for Disease Control and Prevention (2006). The National Breast and Cervical Cancer Early Detection Program, 2006 Fact Sheet.

Cerella, J. (1990). Aging and information processing rate. In J.E. Birren and K.W. Schaie (Eds.) Handbook of the psychology of aging (3rd edition). San Diego: Academic Press.

Chalfonte, B.L. and Johnson, M.K. (1996). Feature memory and binding in young and older adults. Memory and Cognition, 24, 403-416.

Chan, C.W., Hon, H.C., Chien, W.T., et al. (2004). Social support and coping in Chinese patients undergoing cancer surgery. Cancer Nurs, 27(3): 230-6.

Chasens, E.R., Umlauf, M.G., Pillion, D.J., et al. (2000). Sleep apnea symptoms, nocturia, and diabetes in African-American community dwelling older adults. J Natl Black Nurses Assoc, 11 (2): 25-33.

Chelliah, A., Burge, M.R. (2004). Hypoglycaemia in elderly patients with diabetes mellitus: causes and strategies for prevention. Drugs Aging, 21 (8): 511-30.

Chen, H., Cantor, A., Meyer, J., et al. (2003). Can older cancer patients tolerate chemotherapy? A prospective pilot study. Cancer, 97 (4): 1107-14.

Chirikos, T.N., Nickel, J.T. (1986). Socioeconomic determinants of continuing functional disablement from chronic disease episodes. Soc Sci Med, 22 (12): 1329-35.

Chockalingam, A., Campbell, N.R., Fodor, J.G. (2006). Worldwide epidemic of hypertension. Can J Cardiol, 22 (7): 553-5.

Chou, K.L., Chi, I. (2005). Functional disability related to diabetes mellitus in older Hong Kong Chinese adults. Gerontology, 51 (5): 334-9.

Christensen, H., Hofer, S.M., Mackinnon, A.J., et al. (2001). Age is no kinder to the better educated: absence of an association investigated using latent growth techniques in a community sample. Psychological Medicine, 31, 15-28.

Christman, K., Muss, H.B., Case, L.D., et al. (1992). Chemotherapy of metastatic breast cancer in the elderly. The Piedmont Oncology Association experience. JAMA, 268 (1): 57-62.

Chu, L.W., Pei, C.K. (1999). Risk factors for early emergency hospital readmission in elderly medical patients. Gerontology, 45 (4): 220-6.

Churchill, L.R. (2005). Age-rationing in health care: flawed policy, personal virtue. Health Care Anal, 13 (2): 137-46.

Cijevschi, C., Mihai, C., Zbranca, E., et al. (2005). Osteoporosis in liver cirrhosis. Rom J Gastroenterol, 14 (4): 337-41.

Cimmino, M.A., Sarzi-Puttini, P., Scarpa, R., et al. (2005). Clinical presentation of osteoarthritis in general practice: determinants of pain in Italian patients in the AMICA study. Semin Arthritis Rheum, 35 (1 Suppl 1): 17-23.

Clark, F., Azen, S.P., Zemke, R., et al. (1997). Occupational therapy for independent-living older adults. JAMA, 278 (16): 1321-6.

Clark, N.M., Dodge, J.A. (1999). Exploring self-efficacy as a predictor of disease management. Health Educ Behav, 26 (1): 72-89.

Clark, N.M, Janz, N.K., Becker, M.H., et al. (1992). Impact of self-management education on the functional health status of older adults with heart disease. Gerontologist, 32 (4): 438-43.

Clark, W. (1999). The biological basis of aging and death. New York: Oxford U. Press.

Clarkson-Smith, L. and Hartley, A.A. (1989). Relationships between physical exercise and cognitive abilities in older adults. Psychology and Aging, 4, 183-189.

Clarkson-Smith, T.A. and Hartley, A.A. (1990). Structural equation models of relationships between exercise and cognitive abilities. Psychology and Aging, 5, 437-446.

Cleveland Clinic (2003). A Vicious cycle: chronic illness and depression.

ClinicalTrials.gov. Effects of electrical acupuncture and exercise in older adults with chronic low back pain. http://www.clinicalrials.gov/show/ NCT00101387.

Cohen, M., Gensini, G.F., Maritz, F., et al. (2005). The role of gender and other factors as predictors of not receiving reperfusion therapy and of outcome in ST-segment eleation myocardial infarction. J Thromb Thrombolysis, 19 (3): 155-61.

Cohen, S. (2004). Social relationships and health. Amer Psychologist, 59, 676-684.

Colleau, Sophie M. Pain in the elderly with cancer. http://www.whocancerpain.wisc.edu/eng/13_2/pain.html

Cole, C.S. and Tak, S.H. (2006). Assessment of attention in Alzheimer's disease. Geriatric Nursing, 27, 238-243.

Colorectal Cancer Collaborative Group (2000). Surgery for colorectal cancer in elderly patients: a systematic review. Lancet, 356, 968-974.

Comijs, H.C., Dik, M.G., Aartsen, S.J., et al. (2005). The impact of change in cognitive functioning and cognitive decline on disability, well-being, and use of healthcare services in older persons. Dementia and Geriatr Cogn Disorders, 19, 316-323.

Cooper, C., Westlake, S., Harvey, N., et al. (2006). Review: developmental origins of osteoporotic fracture. Osteoporos Int, 17 (3): 337-47.

Costa, P.T. and McCrae, R.R. (1994). Set like plaster: Evidence for the stability of adult personality. In T.F. Heatherton & J.L. Weinberger (Eds.) Can personality change? (pp. 21-40). Washington D.C.: American Psychological Association.

Crofford, L.J., Rowbotham, M.C., Mease, P.J., et al. (2005). Pregabalin for the treatment of fibromyalgia syndrome: results of a randomized, double-blind, placebo-controlled trial. Arthritis Rheum, 52 (4): 1264-73.

Crogan, N. and Pasvogel, A. (2003). The Influence of protein-calorie malnutrition on quality of life in nursing homes. J Ger Series A: Bio Sci Med Sci, 58: 159-164.

Cronan, T.A., Serber, E.R., Walen, H.R., et al. (2002). The influence of age on fibromyalgia symptoms. J Aging Health, 14 (3): 370-84.

Crooks, V.C., Buckwalter, J.G., Petitti, D.B. (2003). Diabetes mellitus and cognitive performance in older women. Ann Epidemiol, 13 (9): 613-9.

Crowther, M., Parker, M., Achenvbaum, W.A., et al. (2002). Rowe and Kahn's model of successful aging revisited. The Gerontologist, 42: 613-620.

Cummings, S.R., Nevitt, M.C., Browner, W.S., et al. (1995). Risk factors for hip fracture in white women. Study of Osteoporotic Fractures Research Group. NEJM, 332: 767-773.

Curry, L.C., Walker, C., Hogstel, M.O., et al. (2005). Teaching older adults to self-manage medications: preventing adverse drug reactions. J Gerontol Nurs, 31 (4): 32-42.

D'Astolfo, C.J., Humphreys, B.K. (2006). A record review of reported musculoskeletal pain in an Ontario long term care facility. BMC Geriatr, 6 (1): 5.

Dajczman, E., Fu, L.Y., Small, D., et al. (1996). Treatment of small cell lung carcinoma in the elderly. Cancer, 77 (10): 2032-8.

Daly, D.D., Carr, L. (2004) Osteoporosis. Screening & treatment for the elderly. Patient Safety & Quality HealthCare, http://www.psqh.com/julsep04/dalycarr.html

Daly, R.M., Brown, M., Bass, S., et al. (2006). Calcium- and vitamin D3-fortified milk reduces bone loss at clinically relevant skeletal sites in older men: a 2-year randomized controlled trial. J Bone Miner Res, 21 (3): 397-405.

Daviglus, M.L., Kiang, L., Pirzada, A., et al. (2003). Favorable cardiovascular risk profile in middle age and health-related quality of life in older age. Arch Internal Med, 163: 2460-2468.

Daviglus, M.L., Kiang, L., Pirzada, A., et al. (2003). Body mass index in middle age and health-related quality of life in older age. Arch Internal Med, 163: 2448-2455.

De Berardis, G., Pellegrini, F., Franciosi, M., et al. (2005). Are Type 2 diabetic patients offered adequate foot care? The role of physician and patient characteristics. J Diab Complic, 19 (6): 319-27.

deBeurs, E., Twish, J.W., Sonnenberg, C., et al. (2005). Stability and change of emotional functioning in late life: modeling of vulnerability profiles. J Affect Dis, 84 (1), 53-62.

De Graaf, E.J., Doornebosch, P.G., Stassen, L.P., et al. (2002). Transanal endoscopic microsurgery for rectal cancer. Eur J Cancer, 38, 904-910.

De Groot, M., Anderson, M., Freedland, K., et al. (2001). Association of depression and diabetes complications: a meta-analysis. Psychosom Med, 63, 619-630.

De Mendonca, A., Ribeiro, F., Guerreiro, M., et al. (2005). Clinical significance of sub cortical vascular disease in patients with mild cognitive impairment. Euro J Neuro, 12, 125-130.

De Nicola, L., Minutolo, R., Gallo, C., et al. (2005). Management of hypertension in chronic kidney disease: the Italian multicentric study. J Nephrol, 18 (4): 397-404.

de Rekeneire, N., Rooks, R.N., Simonsick, E.M., et al. (2003). Racial differences in glycemic control in a well-functioning older diabetic population: findings from the Health, Aging, and Body Composition Study. Diab Care, 26 (7): 1986-92.

Del Aguila, M.A., Reiber, G.E., Koepsell, T.D. (1994). How does provider and patient awareness of high-risk status for lower-extremity amputation influence foot-care practice? Diab Care, 17 (9): 1050-4.

De Leo, D. and Spathonis, K. (2003). Suicide and euthanasia in late life. Aging Clin Exper Res, 15 (2), 99-110.

Dellasega, C. (1990). Self-care for the elderly diabetic. J Gerontol Nurs, 16 (1): 16-20.

Del Rincon, I., Freeman, G.L., Haas, R.W., et al. (2005). Relative contribution of cardiovascular risk factors and rheumatoid arthritis clinical manifestations to atherosclerosis. Arthritis Rheum, 52 (11): 3413-23.

Den Heijer, T., Vermeer, S.E., van Dijk, E.J., et al. (2003). Type 2 diabetes and atrophy of medial temporal lobe structures on brain MRI. Diabetologia, 46 (12): 1604-10. Epub 2003 Nov. 1.

Dennis, N.A., Daselaar, S. and Cabeza. R. (2006). Effects of aging on transient and sustained successful memory encoding activity. Neurobio Aging, Aug. 17.

Dennis, N. A., Howard, J.H. and Howard, D.V. (2006). Implicit sequence learning without motor sequencing in young and old adults. Exper Brain Res, June 20.

Diabetic-Lifestyle.com. Back pain and exercise. http://www.diabetic-lifestyle.com/articles/nov99_burni_1.htm

Di Maio, M., Perrone, F. (2003). Quality of life in elderly patients with cancer. Health Qual Life Outcomes, 1 (1): 44.

Dionne, C.E., Dunn, K.M., Croft, P.R. (2006). Does back pain prevalence really decrease with increasing age? A systematic review. Age Ageing, Mar 17.

Dixon, R.A., Wahlin, A., Maitland, S.B., et al. (2004). Episodic memory change in late adulthood: generalizability across samples and performance indices. Neuropsychology, 19, 768-778.

Doolan, D.M., Froelicher, E.S. (2006). Efficacy of smoking cessation intervention among special populations: review of the literature from 2000 to 2005.

Doran, MF., Crowson, C.S., Pond, G.R., et al. (2002). Predictors of infection in rheumatoid arthritis. Arthritis Rheum, 46 (9): 2294-300.

Dreicer, R., Cooper, C.S., Williams, R.D. (1996). Management of prostate and bladder cancer in the elderly. Urol Clin North Am, 23 (1): 87-97.

Dumont, C.J., Keeling, A.W., Bourguignon, C., et al. (2006). Predictors of vascular complications post diagnostic cardiac catheterization and percutaneous coronary interventions. Dimens Crit Care Nurs, 25 (3): 137-42.

Duverne, S., Lemaire, P. and Vandierendonck, A. (2006). Do working memory executive components mediate the effects of age on strategy selection or on strategy execution? Insights from arithmetic problem solving. Psychological Research, July 13.

Dye, C.J., Haley-Zitlin, V., Willoughby, D. (2003). Insights from older adults with type 2 diabetes: making dietary and exercise changes. Diabetes Educ, 29 (1): 116-27.

Dykes, P.C., Acevedo, K., Boldrighini, J., et al. (2005). Clinical practice guideline adherence before and after implementation of the HEARTFELT (HEART Failure Effectiveness & Leadership Team) intervention. J Cardiovasc Nurs, 20 (5): 306-14.

Eason, S.L., Petersen, N.J., Suarez-Almazor, M., et al. (2005). Diabetes mellitus, smoking, and the risk for asymptomatic peripheral arterial disease: whom should we screen? J Am Board Fam Pract, 18 (5): 355-61.

Edelson, E. (2006). Experts: Screen most older adults to prevent heart attacks. Panel advises regular arterial exams for even healthy Americans. Health on the Net Foundation. http://www.hon.ch/News/HSN/533686.html

Ehrlich, G.E. (2003). Back pain. J Rheumatol Suppl, 67: 26-31.

Elhendy, A., Hamby, R.I., Perry-Bottinger, L. (2006). Heart attacks and women. http://heart.healthcentersonline.com/cholesterol/hrattack women.cfm.

Emanuel, E.J., Fairclough, D.L., Daniels, E.R., et al. (1996). Euthanasia and physician-assisted suicide: attitudes and experiences of oncology patients, oncologists, and the public. Lancet, 347 (9018): 1805-10.

Emery, P., Kosinski, M., Li, T., et al. (2006a). Treatment of rheumatoid arthritis patients with abatacept and methotrexate significantly improved health-related quality of life. J Rheumatol, 33 (4): 681-9.

Emery P., Fleischmann, R., Filipowicz-Sosnowska, A., et al. (2006b). The efficacy and safety of rituximab in patients with active rheumatoid arthritis despite methotrexate treatment: results of a phase IIB randomized, double-blind, placebo-controlled, dose-ranging trial. Arthritis Rheum, 54(5): 1390-400.

Eng, J., Ramsum, D., Verhoef, M., et al. (2003). A population-based survey of complementary and alternative medicine use in men recently diagnosed with prostate cancer. Integr Cancer Ther, 2 (3): 212-6.

Engle, R. W., Kane, M.J. and Tuholski, S.W. (1999). Individual differences in working memory capacity and what they tell us about controlled attention, general fluid intelligence and the functions of the prefrontal cortex. In A. Miyake and P. Shah (Eds.), Models of working memory: Mechanisms of active maintenance and executive control. New York: Cambridge University Press.

Engle, V.F., Graney, M.J., Chan, A. (2001). Accuracy and bias of licensed practical nurse and nursing assistant ratings of nursing home residents' pain. J Ger Series A: Biol Sci Med Sci, 56: M405-M411.

Epstein, S. (2006). Update of current therapeutic options for the treatment of postmenopausal osteoporosis. Clin Ther, 28 (2): 151-73.

Evans, R.I. (2001). Social influences in etiology and prevention of smoking and other health threatening behaviors. In A. Baum, T.A. Revenson and J.E. Singer (Eds.), Handbook of health psychology (pp. 459-468). Mahwah, N.J.: Lawrence Erlbaum Associates.

Fabiani, M., Low, K.A., Sable, J.J., et al. (2006). Reduced suppression or labile memory? Mechanisms of inefficient filtering of irrelevant information in older adults. J Cognitive Neurosci, 18, 637-650.

Farias, S.T., Mungas, D. and Jagust, W. (2005). Degree of discrepancy between self and other-reported everyday functioning by cognitive status: dementia, mild cognitive impairment and healthier adults. Int J Ger Psychiatry, 20, 827-834.

Fattirolli, F., Burgisser, C., Guarducci, L., et al. (2005). Cardiac rehabilitation in the elderly. Ital Heart J Suppl, 6 (12): 788-95.

Faulkner, K.A., Cauley, J.A., Zmuda, J.M., et al. (2005). Ethnic differences in the frequency and circumstances of falling in older community-dwelling women. J Amer Geriatr Soc, 53 (10): 1774-9.

Federal Interagency Forum on Aging-Related Statistics (2004). Older Americans 2004: key indicators of well-being. http://www.agingstats.gov/chartbook2004/healthstatus.html

Federman, AD., Adams, A.S., Ross-Degnan, D., et al. (2001). Supplemental insurance and use of effective cardiovascular drugs among elderly Medicare beneficiaries with coronary heart disease. JAMA, 286 (14): 1762-3.

Felson, D.T., Lawrence, R.C., Dieppe, P.A., et al. (2000). Osteoarthritis: new insights. Part 1: the disease and its risk factors (Consensus Development Conference). Ann Intern Med, 133: 635-646.

Feldstein, A., Elmer, P.J., Smith, D.H., et al. (2006). Electronic medical record reminder improves osteoporosis management after a fracture: a randomized controlled trial. J Am Geriatr Soc, 54 (3): 450-7.

Felton, B.J., Revenson, T.A. (1987). Age differences in coping with chronic illness. Psychol Aging, 2 (2): 164-70.

Ferrara, N., Corbi, G., Bosimini, E., et al. (2006). Cardiac rehabilitation in the elderly: patient selection and outcomes. Am J Geriatr Cardiol, 15 (1): 22-7.

Fick, D.M., Cooper, J.W., Wade, W.E., et al. (2003). Updating the Beers criteria for potentially inappropriate medication use in older adults: results of a US consensus panel of experts. Arch Intern Med, 163 (22): 2716-24.

Ficorella, C., Cannita, K., Ricevuto, E. (1999). The adjuvant therapy of colonic carcinoma in old age. Minerva Med, 90, 232-233.

Fiori, K.L., Hays, J.C., Meador, K.G. (2004). Spiritual turning points and perceived control over the life course. Int J Aging Hum Dev, 59 (4): 391-420.

Firdaus, M., Mathe, M.K., Wright, J. (2006). Health promotion in older adults: the role of lifestyle in the metabolic syndrome. Geriatrics, 61 (2): 18-22, 24-5.

Fishbain, D.A. (1999). The association of chronic pain and suicide. Sem Clin Neuropsych, 4 (3), 221-227.

Fishbain, D.A., Goldberg, M., Rosomoff, R.S., et al. (1991). Completed suicide in chronic pain. Clin J Pain, 7 (1), 29-36.

Fisher, B.J., Haythornthwaite, J.A., Heinberg, L.J., et al. (2001). Suicidal intent in patients with chronic pain. Pain, 89 (2-3), 199-206.

Fisher, D.L. and Glaser, R.A. (1996). Molar and latent models of cognitive slowing: implications for aging, dementia, depression, development and intelligence. Psychonomic Bull Rev, 3, 458-480.

Fleischman, D.A., Wilson, R.S., Gabrieli, J.D., et al. (2005). Implicit memory and Alzheimer's disease neuropathology. Brain, 128, 2006-2015.

Fleischmann, K.E., Orav, E.J., Lamas, G.A., et al. (2006). Pacemaker implantation and quality of life in the Mode Selectio Trial (MOST). Heart Rhythm, 3 (6): 653-9.

Focht, B.C., Rejeski, W.J., Ambrosius, W.T., et al. (2005). Exercise, self-efficacy, and mobility performance in overweight and obese older adults with knee osteoarthritis. Arthritis Rheum, 53 (5): 659-65.

Fontaine, K.R., Haaz, S. (2006). Risk factors for lack of recent exercise in adults with self-reported, professionally diagnosed arthritis. J Clin Rheumatol, 12 (2): 66-9.

Forjuoh, S.N., Reis, M.D., Couchman, G.R., et al. (2005). Physician response to written feedback on a medication discrepancy found with their elderly ambulatory patients. J Am Geriatr Soc, 53 (12): 2173-7.

Fox, P.L., Raina, P., Jadad, A.R. (1999). Prevalence and treatment of pain in older adults in nursing homes and other long-term care institutions: a systematic review. CMAJ, 160 (3): 329-333.

Fox, S.A., Stein, J.A., Sockloskie, R.J., et al. (2001). Targeted mailed materials and the Medicare beneficiary: increasing mammogram screening among the elderly. Am J Public Health, 91 (1): 55-61.

Franck, W.M., Moorahrend, U., Inselmann, U. (2005). Joint replacement surgery in the elderly patient: where to draw the line for the indication? MMW Fortschr Med, 147 (49-50): 44, 46, 48.

Franklin, S.S. (2006). Hypertension in older people. Part 1. J Clin Hypertens (Greenwich), 8 (6): 444-9.

Friedlander, M.A., Hricik, D.E. (1997). Optimizing end-stage renal disease therapy for the patient with diabetes mellitus. Semin Nephrol, 17 (4): 331-45.

Friedman, H.S., Tucker, J.S., Tomlinson-Kearsey, C., et al. (1993). Does childhood personality predict longevity? J Per Soc Psych, 65, 176-185.

Fu, M.R. (2005). Breast cancer survivors' intentions of managing lymphedema. Cancer Nurs, 28 (6): 446-57.

Gabbay, R.A., Lendel, I., Saleem, T.M., et al. (2006). Nurse case management improves blood pressure, emotional distress and diabetes complication screening. Diab Res Clin Pract, 71 (1): 28-35.

Gabriel, S. and Bowling A. (2004). Quality of life from the perspectives of older people. Aging and Society, 24: 675-691.

Gabriel, S.E., Crowson, C.S., Kremers, H.M., et al. (2003). Survival in rheumatoid arthritis: a population-based analysis of trends over 40 years. Arthritis Rheum, 48 (1): 54-8.

Gabriel, S.E., Crowson, C.S., O'Fallon, W.M. (1999). Comorbidity in arthritis. J Rheumatol, 26 (11): 2475-9.

Gage, B.F., Birman-Deych, E., Radford, M.J., et al. (2006). Risk of osteoporotic fracture in elderly patients taking warfarin: results from the National Registry of Atrial Fibrillation 2. Arch Intern Med, 166 (2): 241-6.

Gaglia, J.L., Wyckoff, J., Abrahamson, M.J. (2004). Acute hyperglycemic crisis in the elderly. Med Clin North Am, 88 (4): 1063-84, xii.

Ganz, D.A., Chang, J.T., Roth, C.P., et al. (2006). Quality of osteoarthritis care for community-dwelling older adults. Arthritis Rheum, 55 (2): 241-7.

Ganz, P.A., Guadagnoli, E., Landrum, M.B., et al. (2003). Breast cancer in older women: quality of life and psychosocial adjustment in the 15 months after diagnosis. J Clin Oncol, 21 (21): 4027-33.

Gary, R. (2006). Self-care practices in women with diastolic heart failure. Heart Lung, 35 (1): 9-19.

Gass, M., Dawson-Hughes, B. (2006). Preventing osteoporosis-related fractures: an overview. Am J Med, 119 (4 Suppl 1): S3-S11.

Gavard, J.A., Lustman, P.J., and Clouse, R.E. (1993). Prevalence of depression in adults with diabetes: an epidemiological evaluation. Diab Care 16, 1167-1178.

Genovese, M.C., Becker, J.C., Schiff, M., et al. (2005). Abatacept for rheumatoid arthritis refractory to tumor factor alpha inhibition. NEJM, 353 (11): 1114-23.

Giangregorio, L., Papaioannou, A., Cranney, A., et al. (2006). Fragility fractures and the osteoporosis care gap: an international phenomenon. Semin Arthritis Rheum, 35 (5): 293-305.

Gilden, J.L., Hendryx, M.S., Casia, C., et al. (1989). The effectiveness of diabetes education programs for older patients and their spouses. J Am Geriatr Soc, 37 (11): 1023-30.

Gilden, J.L., Hendryx, M.S., Clar, S., et al. (1992). Diabetes support groups improve health care of older diabetic patients. J Am Geriatr Soc, 40 (2): 147-50.

Giltay, E.J., Geleijnse, J.M., Zitman, F.G., Hoekstra, T. and Schouten, E.G. (2004). Dispostional optimism and all-cause and cardiovascular mortality in a prospective cohort of elderly Dutch men and women, Arch Gen Psychiatry, 61, 1126-1135.

Given, B., Given, C., Azzouz, F., et al. (2001). Physical functioning of elderly cancer patients prior to diagnosis and following initial treatment. Nurs Res, 50 (4): 222-32.

Given, B., Sherwood, P.R. (2006). Family care for the older person with cancer. Semin Oncol Nurs, 22 (1): 43-50.

Glajchen, M. (2004). The emerging role and needs of family caregivers in cancer care. J Support Oncol, 2 (2): 145-55.

Glassman, A. and Shapiro, P. (1998). Depression and the course of coronary artery disease. Amer J Psych, 155, 4-11.

Golby, A., Silverberg, G., Race, E., et al. (2005). Memory encoding in Alzheimer's disease: an MRI study of explicit and implicit memory. Brain, 128, 773-787.

Goldenberg, D.L., Burckhardt, C., Crofford, L. (2004). Management of fibromyalgia syndrome. JAMA, 292 (19): 2388-95.

Goldstein, N.E., Concato, J., Fried, T.R., et al. (2004). Factors associated with caregiver burden among caregivers of terminally ill patients with cancer. J Palliat Care, 20 (1): 38-43.

Gonzales, G.R. (1995). Central pain: diagnosis and treatment strategies. Neurology, 45 (12), 35-36.

Gonzalez, B., Lupon, J., Parajon, T., et al. (2004). Nurse evaluation of patients in a new multidisciplinary Heart Failure Unit in Spain. Eur J Cardiovasc Nurs, 3 (1): 61-9.

Gonzalez, Q.H., Heslin, M.J., Shore, G., et al. (2003). Results of long-term follow-up for transanal excision for rectal cancer. Am Surg, 69, 675-678.

Gonzalez-Gay, M.A., De Matias, J.M., Gonzalez-Juanatey, C., et al. (2006). Anti-tumor necrosis factor-alpha blockade improves insulin resistance in patients with rheumatoid arthritis. Clin Exp Rheumatol, 24 (1): 83-6.

Gott, M., Barnes, S., Parker, C., et al. (2006). Predictors of the quality of life of older people with heart failure recruited from primary care. Age Ageing, 35 (2): 172-7.

Goulding, M.R. (2004). Inappropriate medication prescribing for elderly ambulatory care patients. Arch Intern Med, 164 (3): 305-12.

Gowin, K.M. (2000). Diffuse pain syndromes in the elderly. Rheum Dis Clin North Am, 26 (3): 673-82.

Goya Wannamethee, S., Gerald Shaper, A., Whincup, P.H., et al. (2004). Overweight and obesity and the burden of disease and disability in elderly men. Int J Obes Relat Metab Disord, 28 (11): 1374-82.

Grady, C.L., Springer, M.V., Hongwanishkul, D., et al. (2006). Age-related changes in brain activity across the adult lifespan. J Cognitive Neurosci, 18, 2227-41.

Graybiel, A.M. (2000). The basal ganglia. Current Biol, 10, R509-R511.

Grazio, S., Korsic, M., Jajic, I. (2005). Prevalence of vertebral fractures in an urban population in Croatia aged fifty and older. Wien Klin Wochenschr, 117 (1-2): 42-7.

Green, D.A. (1986). Acute and chronic complications of diabetes mellitus in older patients. Am J Med, 80 (5A): 39-53.

Greene, D.A., Stevens, M.J., Feldman, E.L. (1999). Diabetic neuropathy. Scope of the syndrome. Am J Med, 107: 2S-8S.

Gridelli, C. (2002). Does chemotherapy have a role as palliative therapy for unfit or elderly patients with non-small-cell lung cancer? Lung Cancer, 38 (Suppl 2): S45-50.

Gridelli, C., Aapro, M., Ardizzoni, A., et al. (2005). Treatment of advanced non-small-cell lung cancer in the elderly: results of an international expert panel. J Clin Oncol, 23 (13): 3125-37.

Griffin, K.W., Friend, R., Kaell, A.T. (2001). Distress and disease status among patients with rheumatoid arthritis: roles of coping styles and perceived responses from support providers. Ann Behav Med, 23 (2): 133-8.

Griffin, M.R., Brandt, K.E., Liang, M.H., et al. (1995). Practical management of osteoarthritis. Integration of pharmacologic and nonpharmacologic measures. Arch Fam Med, 4 (12): 1049-55.

Gustafsson, T.M., Isacson, D.G., Thorslund, M. (1998). Mortality in elderly men and women in a Swedish municipality. Age Ageing. 27 (5): 585-93.

Guyton, A.C. and Hall, J.E. (1996). Textbook of medical physiology (9th edition). Philadelphia: Saunders.

Hadjistavropoulos, H.D., Asmundson, G.J., LaChapelle, D.L., et al. (2002). The role of health anxiety among patients with chronic pain in determining response to therapy. Pain Res Manage, 7 (3), 127-133.

Haley, W.E. (2003). Family caregivers of elderly patients with cancer: understanding and minimizing the burden of care. J Support Oncol, 1 (4 Suppl 2): 25-9.

Han, S.Y., Yoon, J.W., Jo, S.K., et al. (2002). Insomnia in diabetic hemodialysis patients. Prevalence and risk factors by a multicenter study. Nephron, 92 (1): 127-32.

Hansberry, M.R., Whittier, W.L., Krause, M.W. (2005). The elderly patient with chronic kidney disease. Adv Chronic Kidney Dis, 12 (1): 71-7.

Hartvigsen, J., Christiansen, K., Frederiksen, H. (2004). Back and neck pain exhibit many common features in old age: a population-based study of 4,486 Danish twins 70-102 years of age. Spine, 29 (5): 576-80.

Hashimoto, A., Sato, H., Nishibayahi, Y., et al. (2001). A multicenter cross-sectional study on the Health Related Quality of Life of patients with rheumatoid arthritis using a revised Japanese version of the Arthritis Impact Measurement Scales Version 2 (AIMS 2), focusing on physical disability and its associative factors. Ryumachi, 41 (1): 9-24.

Hasserius, R., Karlsson, M.K., Jonsson, B., et al. (2005). Long-term morbidity and mortality after a clinically diagnosed vertebral fracture in the elderly—a 12- and 22-year follow-up of 257 patients. Calcif Tissue Int, 76 (4): 235-42.

Hasslacher, C., Wittmann, W. (2003). Severe hypoglycemia in diabetics with impaired renal function. Dtsch Med Wochenschr, 128 (6): 253-6.

Hedden, T. and Gabrieli, J.D. (2005). Healthy and pathological processes in adult development: new evidence from neuroimaging of the aging brain. Current Opin Neurology, 18, 740-747.

Heer, T., Schiele, R., Schneider, S., et al. (2002). Gender differences in acute myocardial infarction in the era of reperfusion (the MITRA registry). Am J Cardiol, 89 (5): 511-7.

Heisler, M., Piette, J.D. (2005). "I help you, and you help me": facilitated telephone peer support among patients with diabetes. Diab Educ, 31 (6): 869-79.

Helfand, A.E. (2003). Assessing and preventing foot problems in older patients who have diabetes mellitus. Clin Podiatr Med Surg, 20 (3): 573-82.

Helmes, E., Bush, J.D., Pike, P.L., et al. (2006). Gender differences in performance of script analysis by older adults. Brain Cognition, June 13.

Helson, R., Jones, C.J., and Kwan, S.Y. (2002). Personality change over 40 years of adulthood: Hierarchical linear modeling analyses of two longitudinal samples. J Per Soc Psych, 83, 752-766.

Henry, J. D., MacLeod, M. S., Phillips, L.H., et al. (2004). A meta-analytic review of prospective memory and aging. Psychology and Aging, 19, 27-39.

Heriot, A.G., Tekkis, P.P., Smith, J.J. (2006). Prediction of postoperative mortality in elderly patients with colorectal cancer. Dis Colon Rectum, 49 (6): 816-24.

Herpertz, S., Johann, B., Lichtblau, K., et al. (2000). Patients with diabetes mellitus: psychosocial stress and use of psychosocial support: a multicenter study. Med Klin (Munich), 95 (7): 369-77.

Herrlinger, C., Klotz, U. (2001). Drug metabolism and drug interactions in the elderly. Best Pract Res Clin Gastroenterol, 15 (6): 897-918.

Hileman, J.W., Lackey, N.R., Hassanein, R.S. (1992). Identifying the needs of home caregivers of patients with cancer. Oncol Nurs Forum, 19 (5): 771-7.

Ho, P., Law, W.L., Chan S.C., et al. (2003). Functional outcome following low anterior resection with total mesorectal excision in the elderly. Int J Colorectal Dis, 18, 230-233.

Hochberg, M.C., Altman, R.D., Brandt, K.D., et al. (1995a). Guidelines for the medical management of osteoarthritis. Part I. Osteoarthritis of the hip. Arthritis Rheum, 38 (11): 1535-40.

Hochberg, M.C., Altman, R.D., Brandt, K.D., et al. (1995b). Guidelines for the medical management of osteoarthritis. Part II. Osteoarthritis of the knee. Arthritis Rheum, 38 (11): 1541-6.

Hogan, P., Dall, T., Nikolov, P. (2003). Economic costs of diabetes in the US in 2002. Diabetes Care, 26 (3): 917-32.

Holland, N.W., Gonzalez, E.B. (1998). Soft tissue problems in adults. Clin Geriatr Med, 14 (3): 601-11.

Hollander, P., Nicewander, D., Couch, C., et al. (2005). Quality of care of Medicare patients with diabetes in a metropolitan fee-for-service primary car integrated delivery system. Am J Med Qual, 20 (6): 344-52.

Holman, H., Lorig, K. (1997). Overcoming barriers to successful aging: self-management of osteoarthritis. West J Med, 167 (4): 265-8.

Holstein, A., Egberts, E.H. (2003). Risk of hypoglycemia with oral anti-diabetic agents in patients with Type 2 diabetes. Exp Clin Endocrinol Diabetes, 111 (7): 405-14.

Honecker, F., Kohne, C.H., Bokemeyer, C. (2003). Colorectal cancer in the elderly: is palliative chemotherapy of value? Drugs Aging, 20 (1): 1-11.

Hootman, J.M., Helmick, C.G. (2006). Projections of US prevalence of arthritis and associated activity limitations. Arthritis Rheum, 54 (1): 226-9.

Hornick, T.R. (2006). Surgical innovations: impact on the quality of life of the older patient. Clin Geriatr Med, 22 (3): 499-513.

Houldin, A.D., Wasserbauer, N. (1996). Psychosocial needs of older cancer patients: a pilot study abstract. Medsurg Nurs, 5 (4): 253-6.

http://www.healthcentral.com/heart-disease/surviving-heartattack-000013_5-145_pf.html, Heart failure-complications.

http://www.merck.com/mmhe/print/sec03/ch033/ch033c.html, Heart attack.

Hu, W.Y., Chiu, T.Y., Chuang, R.B., et al. (2002). Solving family-related barriers to truthfulness in cases of terminal cancer in Taiwan. A professional perspective.

Huh, H.T., Gazzeley, A. and Delis, D.C. (2006). Response bias and aging on a recognition memory task. J Inter Neuropsychology Sociology, 12, 1-7.

Hurria, A., Gupta, S., Zauderer, M., et al. (2005). Developing a cancer-specific geriatric assessment: a feasibility study. Cancer, 104 (9): 1998-2005.

Iki, M., Saito, Y., Kajita, E., et al. (2006). Trunk muscle strength is a strong predictor of bone loss in postmenopausal women. Clin Orthop Relat Res, 443: 66-72.

International Diabetes Federation (2006). Diabetes prevalence. http://www.idf.org/home/index.cfm?node=264.

Iowa Prostate Cancer Consensus Recommendations Committee. The Iowa prostate cancer consensus: Screening and management in men aged 75 years of age and older.

Isbister, W.H. (1997). Colorectal surgery in the elderly: an audit of surgery in octogenarians. Aust N Z Surg, 67 (8): 557-61.

Ishida, Y., Kawai, S., Taguchi, T. (2005). Factors affecting ambulatory status and survival of patients 90 years and older with hip fractures. Clin Orthop Relat Res, (436): 208-15.

Ishii, H. (2006). Caring for elderly patients with diabetes by understanding psychological status. Nippon Rinsho, 64 (1): 128-33.

Ismail, A.A., Cooper, C., Felsenberg, D., et al. (1999). Number and type of vertebral deformities: epidemiological characteristics and relation to back pain and height loss. European Vertebral Osteoporosis Study Group. Osteoporos Int, 9 (3): 206-13.

Issa, S.N., Sharma, L. (2006). Epidemiology of osteoarthritis: an update. Curr Rheumatol Rep, 8 (1): 7-15.

Iwamoto, J., Takeda, T., Sato, Y. (2006). Efficacy and safety of alendronate and risedronate for postmenopausal osteoporosis. Curr Med Res Opin, 22 (5): 919-28.

Iwasaki, Y., Butcher, J. (2004). Coping with stress among middle-aged and older women and men with arthritis. Int J Psychosoc Rehab, 8, 179-208.

Jaarsma, T., Halfens, R., Huijer Abu-Saad, H., et al. (1999). Effects of education and support on self-care and resource utilization in patients with heart failure. Eur Heart J, 20 (9): 673-82.

Jack, L., Jr., Airhihenbuwa, C.O., Namageyo-Funa, A., et al. (2004). The psychosocial aspects of diabetes care. Using collaborative care to manage older adults with diabetes. Geriatrics, 59 (5): 26-31.

Jackson, J.L., Meyer, G.S., Pettit, T. (2000). Complications from cardiac catheterization: analysis of a military database. Mil Med 165 (4): 298-301.

Jacobs, J.M., Hammerman-Rozenberg, R., Cohen, A., et al. (2006). Chronic back pain among the elderly: prevalence, associations, and predictors. Spine, 31 (7): E203-7.

Jacoby, L.L., Bishara, A.J., Hessels, S., et al. (2005). Aging, subjective experience, and cognitive control: dramatic false remembering by older adults. J Exper Psych: General, 134, 131-148.

Jaklitsch, M.T., Mery, C.M., Audisio, R.A. (2003). The use of surgery to treat lung cancer in elderly patients. Lancet Oncol, 4 (8): 463-71.

Jakobsson, U., Hallberg, I.R. (2002). Pain and quality among older people with rheumatoid arthritis and/or osteoarthritis: a literature review. J Clin Nurs, 11 (4): 430-43.

Jandorf, L., Gutierrez, Y., Lopez, J., et al. (2005). Use of a patient navigator to increase colorectal cancer screening in an urban neighborhood health clinic. J Urban Hlth 82 (2): 216-24.

Jang, Y., Poon, L.W., and Martin, P. (2004). Individual differences in the effects of disease and disability on depressive symptoms: the role of age and subjective health. Int J Aging Hum Dev, 59 (2), 125-137.

Janssen, I., Mark, A.E. (2006). Separate and combined influence of body mass index and waist circumference on arthritis and knee osteoarthritis. Int J Obes (Lond), March 7 (Epub ahead of print).

Jiang, S.L., Ji, X.P., Zhao, Y.X., et al. (2006). Predictors of in-hospital mortality difference between male and female patients with acute myocardial infarction. Am J Cardiol, 98 (8): 1000-3.

Johanna Briggs Institute (2006). Strategies to reduce medication errors with reference to older adults. Nurs Stand, 20 (41): 53-7.

Johnson, J.E. (1996). Sleep problems and self-care in very old rural women. Ger Nurs, 17, 72-74.

Johnson, N.J., Backlund, E., Sorlie, P.D. and Loveless, C.A. (2000). Marital status and mortality: The National Longitudinal Mortality Study. Ann Epidemiol, 10, 224-238.

Jones, C.J., Livson, N. and Peskin, H. (2003). Longitudinal hierarchical linear modeling analyses of California Psychological Inventory data from age 33 to 75: An examination of stability and change in adult personality. J Pers Assess, 80, 294-308.

Kagay, C.R., Quale, C., Smith-Bindman, R. (2006). Screening mammography in the American elderly. Am J Prev Med, 31 (2): 142-9.

Kanaya, A.M., Barrett-Connor, E., Gildengorin, G., et al. (2004). Change in cognitive function by glucose tolerance status in older adults: a 4-year prospective study of the Rancho Bernardo study cohort. Arch Int Med, 164(12): 1327-33.

Kapiteijn, E., van de Velde, C.J. (2002). The role of total mesorectal excision in the management of rectal cancer. Surg Clin North Am, 82, 995-1007.

Kapp, M.B. (2002). Health care rationing affecting older persons: rejected in principle but implemented in fact. J Aging Soc Policy, 14 (2): 27-42.

Karlsen, B., Idsoe, T., Dirdal, I. (2004). Effects of a group-based counseling programme on diabetes-related stress, coping, psychological well-being and metabolic control in adults with type 1 or type 2 diabetes. Patient Educ Couns, 53 (3): 299-308.

Kaski, J.C., Smith, D.A. (2000). The management of chronic ischemic heart disease in the elderly. Am J Geriatr Cardiol, 9 (3): 145-150.

Katon, W., Unutzer, J., Fan, M.Y., et al. (2006). Cost-effectiveness and net benefit of enhanced treatment of depression for older adults with diabetes and depression. Diab Care, 29 (2): 265-70.

Katz, J.N. (2006). Lumbar disc disorders and low-back pain: socioeconomic factors and consequences. J Bone Joint Surg Am, 88 (Suppl 2): 21-4.

Kaufman, S.R., Shim, J.K., Russ, A.J. (2006). Old age, life extension, and the character of medical choice. J Gerontol B Psychol Sci Soc Sci, 61 (4): S175-84.

Kawachi, I., Sparrow, D., Vokonas, P.S. and Weiss, S.T. (1994). Symptoms of anxiety and risk of coronary heart disease: The normative aging study, Circulation, 90, 2225-2229.

Keen, R.W. (2003). Burden of osteoporosis and fractures. Curr Osteoporos Rep, 1 (2): 66-70.

Keller, H.H., Ostbye, T. and Goy, R. (2004) Nutritional risk predicts quality of life in elderly community-living Canadians. J Ger Series A: Bio Sci Med Sci, 59: 68-74.

Kelsey, J.L., Browener, W.S., Seeley, D.G., et al. (1992). Risk factors for fractures of distal forearm and proximal humerus. The Study of Osteoporotic Fractures Research Group. Am J Epidemiol, 135, 477-489.

Kemper, S., Herman, R.E. and Lian, C.H.T. (2003). The costs of doing two things at once for young and older adults: Talking while walking, finger tapping and ignoring speech noise. Psychology and Aging, 18, 181-192.

Kennedy, M., Solomon, C., Manolio, T.A., et al. (2005). Risk factors for declining ankle-brachial index in men and women 65 years or older: the Cardiovascular Health Study. Arch Intern Med, 165 (16): 1896-902.

Keysor, J.J. and Jette, A.M. (2001). Have we oversold the benefit of late-life exercise? J Ger A: Bio Sci Med Sci, 56, 412-423.

Kiecolt-Glaser, J.R., McGuire, L., Robles, T.F. and Glaser, R. (2002). Psychoneuroimmunology: Psychological influences on immune function and health. J Consult Clin Psychology, 70, 537-547.

Kimble, L.P., Kunik, C.L. (2000). Knowledge and use of sublingual nitroglycerin and cardiac-related quality of life in patients with chronic stable angina. J Pain Symptom Manage, 19 (2): 109-17.

Kisley, M.A., Davalos, D.B., Engleman, L.L., et al. (2005). Age-related change in neural processing of time-dependent stimulus features. Brain Res Cognitive Brain Res, 25, 913-925.

Klin Med. (2006). Cerebrovascular disturbances in rheumatoid arthritis. Klin Med, 84 (1): 42-5.

Kloner, R.A. (2004). Assessment of cardiovascular risk in patients with erectile dysfunction: focus on the diabetic patient. Endocrine, 23 (2-3): 125-9.

Knowler, W.C., Barrett-Connor, E., Fowler, S.E., et al. (2002). Reduction in incidence of type 2 diabetes with lifestyle intervention of metformin. NEJM, 346: 393-403.

Koenig, H.G. (2006). Comparison of older depressed hospitalized patients with and without heart failure/pulmonary disease. Aging Ment Health, 10 (4): 335-42.

Koenig, H.G., Cohen, H.J., Blazer, D.G., et al. (1995). Religious coping and cognitive symptoms of depression in elderly medical patients. Psychosomatics, 36 (4): 369-75.

Koenig, H.G., McCullough, M.E. and Larson, D.B. (Eds.) (2001). Handbook of Religion and Health. Oxford: Oxford University Press.

Kohout, M.L., Cooper, M.M., Nickolaus, M.S., et al. (2002). Exercise and psychosocial factors modulate immunity to influenza vaccine in elderly individuals. J Ger: Series A: Bio Sci Med Sci, 57A, M557-M562.

Koizumi, K., Haraguchi, S., Hirata, T., et al. (2002). Video-assisted lobectomy in elderly lung cancer patients. Jpn J Thorac Cardiovasc Surg, 50, 15-22.

Kolh, P., Kerzmann, A., Lahaye, L., et al. (2001). Cardiac surgery in octogenarians; peri-operative outcome and long-term results. Eur Heart J, 22 (14): 1235-43.

Koperna, T., Kisser, M., Schulz, F. (1997). Emergency surgery for colon cancer in the aged. Arch Surg, 132, 1032-1037.

Kornblith, A.B., Herndon, J.E. 2nd, Weiss, R.B., et al. (2003). Long-term adjustment of survivors of early-stage breast carcinoma, 20 years after adjuvant chemotherapy. Cancer, 98 (4): 679-89.

Kosiborod, M., Lichtman, J.H., Heidenreich, P.A., et al. (2006). National trends in outcomes among elderly patients with heart failure. Am J Med, 119 (7): 616. e1-7.

Kostka, T., Berthouze, S.F., Lacour, J., et al. (2000). The symptomatology of upper respiratory tract infections and exercise in elderly people. Med Sci Sports Exerc, 32: 46-51.

Kozanoglu, E., Canataroglu, A., Abayli, B., et al. (2003). Fibromyalgia syndrome in patients with hepatitis C infection. Rheumatol Int, 23 (5): 248-51.

Krantz, N. and McCerney, M.K. (2002). Effects of psychological and social factors on organic disease: A critical assessment of research on coronary heart disease. Ann Rev Psychol, 53, 341-369.

Krause, N. (2004). Religion and mental health. In R. Hummer and C.G. Ellison (Eds.), Religion, family and health. Oxford: Oxford University Press.

Krause, N. (2003). A preliminary assessment of race differences in the relationship between religious doubt and depressive symptoms. Rev Relig Res, 45, 93-115.

Krause, N. and Ellison, C.E. (2003). Forgiveness by God, forgiveness of others, and psychological well-being in late life. J Sci Study Religion, 42, 77-93.

Krishnan, E., Lingala, V.B., Singh, G. (2004). Declines in mortality from acute myocardial infarction in successive incidence and birth cohorts of patients with rheumatoid arthritis. Circulation, 110 (13): 1774-9.

Krishnan, M., Lok, C.E., Jassal, S.V. (2002). Epidemiology and demographic aspects of treated end-stage renal disease in the elderly. Semin Dial, 15 (2): 79-83.

Kristofferson, M.L., Lofmark, R., Carlsson M. (2003). Myocardial infarction: gender differences in coping and social support. J Adv Nurs, 44 (4): 360-74.

Kroot, E.J., van Gestel, A.M., Swinkels, H.L., et al. (2001). Chronic comorbidity in patients with early rheumatoid arthritis: a descriptive study. J Rheumatol, 28 (7): 1511-7.

Kubzansky, L.D., Sparrow, D., Vokonas, P., et al. (2001). Is the glass half empty or half full? A prospective study of optimism and coronary heart disease in the Normative Aging Study, Psychosom Med, 63, 910-916.

Kurlansky, P.A., Williams, D.B., Traad, E.A., et al. (2006). The valve of choice in elderly patients and its influence on quality of life: a long-term comparative study. J Heart Valve Dis, 15 (2): 180-9.

Kurtz, M.E., Kurtz, J.C., Stommel, M., et al. (2002). Predictors of depressive symptomatology of geriatric patients with lung cancer-a longitudinal analysis. Psychooncology, 11 (1): 12-22.

Kyllonen, P.C. (1996). Is working memory capacity Spearman's g? In I. Dennis and P. Tapsfield (Eds.), Human abilities: Their nature and measurement. Mahwah, N.J: Erlbaum.

LaBerge, D. (1995). Attentional Processing. Cambridge, MA: Harvard University Press.

Lacey, E.A., Musgrave, R.J., Freeman, J.V., et al. (2004). Psychological morbidity after myocardial infarction in an area of deprivation in the UK: evaluation of a self-help package. Eur J Cardiovasc Nurs, 3 (3): 219-24.

Langer, C.J. (2002). Elderly patients with lung cancer: biases and evidence. Curr Treat Options Oncol, 3 (1): 85-102.

Latkauskas, T., Rudinskaite, G., Kurtinaitis, J., et al. (2005). The impact of age on post-operative outcomes of colorectal cancer patients undergoing surgical treatment. BMC Cancer, 5, 153.

Lawry, L.W., Conco, D. (2002). Exploring the meaning of spirituality with aging adults in Appalachia. J Holistic Nurs, 20 (4): 388-402.

Lawton, M.P. (1996) Quality of life and affect in later life. In C. Magai and S. McFadden (eds.), A Handbook of Emotion, Adult Development and Aging. San Diego: Academic Press.

Lawton, M.P., Moss, M., Hoffman, C., et al. (1999) Health, valuation of life and the wish to live. Gerontologist, 39: 406-416.

Lebow, J. (1998). Aging: fact and fiction. Fam Ther Networker, 4: 27-33.

Lehto, U.S., Ojanen, M., Dyba, T., et al. (2006). Baseline psychosocial predictors of survival in localised breast cancer. Br J Cancer, 94 (9): 1245-52.

Le Parc, J.M. (2005). Inflammatory arthritis of the elderly. Rev Prat, 55 (19): 2115-20.

Lerman, I.G., Villa, A.R., Martinez, C.L., et al. (1998). The prevalence of diabetes and associated coronary risk factors in urban and rural older Mexican populations. J Am Geriatr Soc, 46 (11): 1387-95.

Lesperance, M.E., Bell, S.E., Ervin, N.E. (2005). Heart failure and weight gain monitoring. Lippincotts Case Manag, 10 (6): 287-93.

Lev, E.L., Paul, D., Owen, S.V. (1999). Age, self-efficacy, and change in patients' adjustment to cancer. Cancer Pract, 7 (4): 170-6.

Leveille, S.G., Bean, J., Bandeen-Roche, K., et al. (2002). Musculoskeletal pain and risk for falls in older disabled women living in the community. J Am Geriatr Soc, 50 (4): 671-8.

Levinson, M.R., Aldwin, C.M., and Spiro, A. (1998). Age, cohort and period effects on alcohol consumption and problem drinking: Findings from the Normative Aging Study. J Stud Alcohol, 59, 712-722.

Li, J., Morcom, A.M. and Rugg, M.D. (2004). The effects of age on the neural correlates of successful episodic retrieval: an ERP study. Cognit, Affect Behav Neurosci, 4, 279-293.

Li, S.C., Naveh-Benjamin, M. and Lindenberger, U. (2005). Aging neuro-modulation impairs associative binding: a neurocomputational account. Psych Sci, 16, 445-450.

Liang, W., Burnett, C.B., Rowland, J.H., et al. (2002). Communication between physicians and older women with localized breast cancer: implications for treatment and patient satisfaction. J Clin Oncol, 20 (4): 1008-16.

Licht-Strunk, F., Bremmer, M.A., van Marwijk, H.W., et al. (2004). Depression in older persons with versus without vascular disease in the open population: similar depressive patterns, more disability. J Affect Disord, 83 (2-3), 155-160.

Lien, M.C., Allen, P.A., Ruthruff, E., et al. (2006). Visual word recognition without central attention: evidence for greater automaticity with advancing age. Psych Aging, 21, 431-447.

Light, L.L., Prull, M.W., La Voie, D.J., et al. (2000). Dual-process theories of memory in old age. In T.J. Perfect and E.A. Maylor (Eds.), Models of cognitive aging. Oxford, England: Oxford University Press.

Liu, S., Song, Y., Ford, E.S., et al. (2005). Dietary calcium, vitamin D, and the prevalence of metabolic syndrome in middle-aged and older U.S. women. Diab Care, 28 (12): 2926-32.

Lock, K., Pomerleau, J., Causer, L., et al. (2005). The global burden of disease attributable to low consumption of fruit and vegetables: implications for the global strategy on diet. Bull World Health Organ, 83 (2): 100-8.

Logminiene, Z., Norkus, A., Valius, L. (2004). Direct and indirect diabetes costs in the world. Medicina, 40 (1): 16-26.

Louis, E.D., Schupf, N., Manly, J., et al. (2005). Association between mild parkinsonian signs and mild cognitive impairment in a community. Neurology, 64, 1157-1161.

Lovheim, H., Sandman, P., Kallin, K., et al. (2006). Poor staff awareness of analgesic treatment jeopardizes adequate pain control in the care of older people. Age Ageing, 35 (3): 257-261.

Luchsinger, J.A., Reitz, C., Honig, L.S., et al. (2005). Aggregation of vascular risk factors and risk of incident Alzheimer disease. Neurology, 65 (4): 545-51.

Lutgendorf, S.K. and Costanzo, E.S. (2003). Psychonuroimmunology and health psychology: An integrative model. Brain, Behav Immun, 17 (4), 225-232.

Lynn, S., Sainsbury, R., Searle, M. (2005). Older patients in the nephrology clinic—should they be referred? N Z Med J, 118 (1225): U1728.

Macfarlane, G.J., McBeth, J., and Silman, A.J. (2001). Widespread body pain and mortality: prospective population based study. Br Med J, 323, 662-665.

Machado, G.M., Barreto, S.M., Passos, V.M., et al. (2006). Health status and indicators among community-dwelling elders with arthritis: the Bambui health and aging study. J Rheumatol, 33 (2): 342-7.

Mackinnon, A., Christensen, H. and Jorm, A.F. (2006). Search for a common cause factor amongst cognitive, speed and biological variables using narrow age cohorts. Gerontology, 52, 243-257.

Mackowiak-Cordoliani, M.A., Bombois, S., Memin, A., et al. (2005). Poststroke dementia in the elderly. Drugs Aging, 22, 483-493.

Macrae, F.A., St. John, D.J., Ambikapathy, A. et al. (1986). Factors affecting compliance in colorectal cancer screening. Results of a study performed in Ballarat. Med J Aust, 144 (12): 621-3.

Magai, C. and McFadden, S. (1996). Handbook of emotion, adult development and aging. San Diego: Academic Press.

Magni, G., Rigatti-Luchini, S., Fracca, F., et al. (1998). Suicidality in chronic abdominal pain: an analysis of the Hispanic Health and Nutrition Examination Survey. Pain, 76 (1-2), 137-144.

Maly, R.C., Leake, B., Silliman, R.A. (2003). Health care disparities in older patients with breast carcinoma: informational support from physicians. Cancer, 97 (6): 1517-27.

Maly, R.C., Umezawa, Y., Leake, B., et al. (2004). Determinants of participation in treatment decision-making by older breast cancer patients. Breast Cancer Res Treat, 85 (3): 201-9.

Maly, R.C., Umezawa, Y., Leake, B., et al. (2005). Mental health outcomes in older women with breast cancer: impact of perceived family support and adjustment. Psychooncology, 14 (7): 535-45.

Maly, R.C., Umezawa, Y., Ratliff, C.T., et al. (2006). Racial/ethnic group differences in treatment decision-making and treatment received among older breast carcinoma patients. Cancer, 106 (4): 957-65.

Managing osteoarthritis: Helping the elderly maintain function and mobility. (3/14/2006) Research in Action, Issue 4, http://www.ahrq.gov/research/osteoria/osteoria.htm.

Manini, T.M., Everhart, J.E., Patel, K.V., et al. (2006). Daily activity energy expenditure and mortality among older adults. JAMA, 296: 171-179.

Manton, K.G., Gu, X. (2001). Changes in the prevalence of chronic disability in the United States black and nonblack population above age 65 from 1982 to 1999. Proceedings of the National Academy of Sciences, 98 (11): 6354-6359.

Maradit-Kremers, H., Crowson, C.S., Nicola, P.J., et al. (2005a). Increased unrecognized coronary heart disease and sudden deaths in rheumatoid arthritis: a population-based cohort study. Arthritis Rheum, 52 (2): 402-11.

Maradit-Kremers, H., Nicola, P.J., Crowson, C.S., et al. (2005b). Cardiovascular death in rheumatoid arthritis: a population-based study. Arthritis Rheum, 52 (3): 722-32.

Maraldi, C., Volpato, S., Kritchevsky, S.B., et al. (2006). Impact of inflammation on the relationship among alcohol consumption, mortality, and cardiac events: the health, aging, and body composition study. Arch Intern Med, 166 (14): 1490-7.

Maravic, M., Le Bihan, C., Landais, P., et al. (2005). Incidence and cost of osteoporotic fractures in France during 2001. A methodological approach by the national hospital database. Osteoporosis Int, 16 (12): 1475-80.

March, L.M., Stenmark, J. (2001). Managing arthritis. Non-pharmacological approaches to managing arthritis. MJA, 175: S102-S107.

Marchionni, N., Fattirolli, F., Fumagilli, S., et al. (2000). Determinants of exercise tolerance after acute myocardial infarction in older persons. J Am Geriatr Soc, 48 (2): 146-53.

Marchionni, N., Fattirolli, F., Fumagalli, S., et al. (2003). Improved exercise tolerance and quality of life with cardiac rehabilitation of older patients after myocardial infarction: results of a randomized, controlled trial. Circulation, 107 (17): 2201-6.

Marin, R., Coca, A., Tranche, S., et al. (2002). Prevalence of renal involvement of type II diabetics followed up in primary care. Nefrologia, 22 (2): 152-61.

Mark, R.E. and Rugg, M.D. (1998). Age effects on brain activity associated with episodic memory retrieval: an electrophysiological study. Brain, 121, 861-873.

Marso, S.P., Hiatt, W.R. (2006). Peripheral arterial disease in patients with diabetes. J Am Coll Cardiol, 47 (5): 921-9. Epub 2006 Feb. 9.

Marzari, C., Maggi, S., Manzato, E., et al. (2005). Depressive symptoms and development of coronary heart disease events: The Italian longitudinal study on aging. J Ger: Bio Med Sci, 60, 85-92.

Masoudi, F.A., Rumsfeld, J.S., Havranek, E.P., et al. (2004). Age, functional capacity, and health-related quality of life in patient with heart failure. J Card Fail, 10 (5): 368-73.

Masoudi, F.A., Baillie, C.A., Wang, Y., et al. (2005). The complexity and cost of drug regimens of older patients hospitalized with heart failure in the United States, 1998-2001. Arch Intern Med, 165 (18): 2069-76.

Matasar, M.J., Sundararajan, V., Grann, V.R., et al. (2004). Management of colorectal cancer in elderly patients: focus on the cost of chemotherapy. Drugs Aging, 21 (2): 113-33.

Matsuoka, K. (2006). Role of diabetes educator for elderly patients. Nippon Rinsho, 64 (1): 149-54.

Mattay, V.S., Fera, F., Tessitore, A., et al. (2006). Neurophysiological correlates of age-related changes in working memory capacity. Neurosci Letter, 392, 32-37.

Maurits, N.M., van der Hoeven, J.H., de Jong, R. (2006). EEG coherence from an auditory oddball task increases with age. Clin Neurophysiol, 23, 395-403.

Maynard, C., Every, N.R., Martin, J.S., et al. (1997). Association of gender and survival in patients with acute myocardial infarction. Arch Int Med, 157 (12): 1379-84.

McArthur Foundation study on aging in America (1998). In J.W. Rowe and R.L. Kahn (Eds.) Successful Aging. New York: Pantheon Books.

McBean, A.M., Shuling, L., Gilbertson, D.T., et al. (2004). Differences in diabetes prevalence, incidence, and mortality among the elderly of four racial/ethnic groups: Whites, Blacks, Hispanics, and Asians. Diab Care, 27: 2317-2324.

McClean, W.J., Higginbotham, N.H. (2002). Prevalence of pain among nursing home residents in rural New South Wales. Med J Aust, 177 (1): 17-20.

McClung, M.R., Siris, E., Cummings, S., et al. (2006). Prevention of bone loss in postmenopausal women treated with lasofoxifene compared with raloxifene. Menopause, May 25.

McCoy, C.B., Anwyl, R.S., Metsch, L.R., et al. (1995). Prostate cancer in Florida: knowledge, attitudes, practices, and beliefs. Cancer Pract, 3 (2): 88-93.

McDougall, G.J. (2004). Memory self-efficacy and memory performance among black and white elders. Nursing Research, 53, 323-331.

McGuire, L.C., Ford, E.S. and Ajani, U.A. (2006). Cognitive functioning as a predictor of functional disability in later life. Amer J Ger Psychiatry, 14, 36-42.

McPhillips, J.B., Barrett-Connor, E., Wingard, D.L. (1990). Cardiovascular disease risk factors prior to the diagnosis of impaired glucose tolerance and non-insulin dependent diabetes mellitus in a community of older adults. Am J Epidemiol, 131 (3): 443-53.

Mehnert, A., Shim, E.J., Koyama, A., et al. (2006). Health-related quality of life in breast cancer: A cross-cultural survey of German, Japanese, and South Korean patients. Breast Cancer Res Treat, May 10.

Mell, T., Heekeren, H.R., Marschner, A., et al. (2005). Effect of aging on stimulus-reward association learning. Neuropsychologia, 43, 554-563.

Meller, S. (2001). A comparison of the well-being of family caregivers of elderly patients hospitalized with physical impairments versus the caregivers of patients hospitalized with dementia. J Am Med Dir Assoc, 2 (2): 60-5.

Mellick, E., Buckwalter, K.C. and Stolley, J.M. (1992). Suicide among elderly white men: development of a profile. J Psychosoc Nurs Mental Hlth Serv, 30 (2), 29-34.

Mellstrom, D., Johnell, O., Ljunggren, O., et al. (2006). Free testosterone is an independent predictor of BMD and prevalent fractures in elderly men: MrOS Sweden. J Bone Miner Res, 21 (4): 529-35.

Menec, V.H. (2003). The relation between everyday activities and successful aging: a 6-year longitudinal study. J Ger Series B: Psycholog Sci Soc Sci, 58: 74-82.

Meyer, K.A., Kushi, L.H., Jacobs, D.R., Jr., et al. (2001). Dietary fat and incidence of type 2 diabetes in older Iowa women. Diab Care 24 (9): 1528-35.

Miazgowski, T. (2005). The prospective evaluation of the osteoporotic vertebral fractures incidence in a random population sample. Endokrynol Pol, 56 (2): 154-9.

Micik, S., Borbasi, S. (2002). Effect of support programme to reduce stress in spouses whose partners 'fall off' clinical pathways post cardiac surgery. Aust Crit Care, 15 (1): 33-40.

Mikuls, T., Saag, K., Criswell, L., et al. (2003). Health related quality of life in women with elderly onset rheumatoid arthritis. J Rheumatol, 30 (5): 952-7.

Mishel, M.H., Germino, B.B., Gil, K.M., et al. (2005). Benefits from an uncertainty management intervention for African-American and Caucasian older long-term breast cancer survivors. Psychooncology, 14 (11): 962-78.

Mitchell, J.L. (1998). Cross-cultural issues in the disclosure of cancer. Cancer Pract, 6 (3): 153-60.

Mitchell, K.J., Johnson, M.K., Raye, C.L., et al. (2000). MRI evidence of age-related hippocampal dysfunction in feature binding in working memory. Cognitive Brain Research, 10, 197-206.

MMWR (1996). Prevalence and impact of arthritis by race and ethnicity– United States, 1989-1991. 45 (18): 373-378.

Monane, M., Matthias, D.M., Nagle, B.A. (1998). Improving prescribing patterns for the elderly through an online drug utilization review inter-vention: a system linking the physician, pharmacist, and computer. JAMA, 280 (14): 1249-52.

Moody-Ayers, S.Y., Stewart, A.L., Covinsky, K.E., et al. (2005). Prevalence and correlates of perceived societal racism in older African-American adults with type 2 diabetes mellitus. J Am Geriatr Soc, 53 (12): 2202-8.

Moore, R., Pedel, S., Lowe, R., et al. (2006). Health-related quality of life following percutaneous coronary intervention: the impact of age on outcome at 1 year. Am J Geriatr Cardiol, 15 (3): 161-4.

Moos, R.H., Schutte, K., Brennan, P., et al. (2004). Ten-year patterns of alcohol consumption and drinking problems among older women and men. Addiction, 99, 829-838.

Morewitz, S. (2006). Chronic Diseases and Health Care. New York: Springer Science+Business Media, Inc.

Morewitz, S. (2004). Marital status as a risk factor for hypertension impairment. (abstract) Circulation, online, 109 (20), p. 89, p. 18.

Morley, J.E. (1998). The elderly type 2 diabetic patients: Special consid-erations. Diabet Med, 1 (Suppl. 4): S41-S46.

Murase, Y., Imagawa, A., Hanafusa, T. (2006). Sick-day management in elderly patients with diabetes mellitus. Nippon Rinsho, 64 (1): 124-7.

Muss, H.B. (1996). Breast cancer in older women. Semin Oncol, 23 (1 Suppl 2): 82-8.

Naghavi, M., Falk, E., Hecht, H.S., et al. (2006). From vulnerable plaque to vulnerable patient—Part III: Executive summary of the Screening for Heart Attack Prevention and Education (SHAPE) Task Force report. Am J Cardiol, 98 (2A): 2H-15H.

Narendran, V., John, R.K., Raghuram, A., et al. (2002). Diabetic retinopa-thy among self reported diabetics in southern India: a population based assessment. Br J Ophthalmol, 86 (9): 1014-8.

Narita, M., Kuzumaki, N., Narita, M., et al. (2006). Age-related emotionality is associated with cortical delta-opoid receptor dysfunction-dependent astrogliosis. Neuroscience, 137 (4), 1359-1367.

National Arthritis Plan (1999) (cited in: About arthritis, http://www.depuyorthopaedics.com/bgdisplayjhtml)

National Center for Health Statistics E Stats (2004). Deaths: Preliminary Data for 2004. USDHHS, Center for Disease Control and Prevention. Hyattsville, MD, http://www.cdc.gov/nchs/products/pubs/pubd/hestats/prelimdeaths04/preliminarydeaths04.

National Fibromyalgia Association (2006). About fibromyalgia & chronic fatigue syndrome. Fibromyalgia fact sheet, http://chronicfatigue.about.com/od/fibromyalgia/a/fmfacts.htm

Naveh-Benjamin, M. (2000). Adult-age differences in memory performance: tests of an associative deficit hypothesis. J Exper Psych: Learning, Memory Cognition, 26, 1170-1187.

Naveh-Benjamin, M. (2001). The effects of divided attention on encoding processes: underlying mechanisms. In M. Naveh-Benjamin, M. Moscovitch and H.L. Roediger (Eds.), Perspectives on human memory and cognitive aging: essays in honour of Fergus Craik. Philadelphia: Psychology Press.

Naveh-Benjamin, M., Hussain, Z., Guez, J., et al. (2003). Adult age differences in episodic memory: further support for an associative-deficit hypothesis. J Exper Psych: Learning, Memory Cognition, 29, 826-837.

Naveh-Benjamin, M., Guez, J., Bilb, A., et al. (2004). The associative memory deficit in older adults: further support using face-name associations. Psych Aging, 19, 541-546.

Naveh-Benjamin, M., Craik, F.I.M., Guez, J., et al. (2005). Divided attention in younger and older adults: effects of strategy and relatedness on memory performance and secondary task costs. J Exper Psych: Learning, Memory Cognition, 31, 520-537.

Newton, J.L., Jones, D.E., Wilton, K., et al. (2006). Calcaneal bone mineral density in older patients who have fallen. QJM, 99 (4): 231-6.

Nicolucci, A., Cavaliere, D., Scorpiglione, N., et al. (1996). A comprehensive assessment of the avoidability of long-term complications of diabetes. A case-control study. SID-AMD Italian Study Group for the Implementation of the St. Vincent Declaration. Diab Care, 19 (9): 927-33.

NIH News Release (1998). Arthritis prevalence rising as baby boomers grow older. Osteoarthritis second only to chronic heart disease in worksite disability. http://www.nih.gov/news/pr/may98/niams-05.htm

Oberauer, K. and Kliegl, R. (2001). Beyond resources: Formal models of complexity effects and age differences in working memory. Euro J Cognitive Psych, 13, 187-215.

Oberauer, K., Wendland, M. and Kliegl, R. (2003). Age differences in working memory: The roles of storage and selective access. Memory Cognition, 31, 563-569.

Olszowska, A., Pietrzak, B., Wankowicz, Z. (2001). Survival of patients with diabetic nephropathy on continuous ambulatory peritoneal dialysis. Own experiences. Pol Arch Med Wewn, 106 (5): 1041-8.

O'Malley, N.C. (assisted by S. Morewitz and G. Knox). Age-based rationing of health care: a descriptive survey of professional attitudes. Health Care Managem Rev, Winter 1991, 16 (1): 83-93.

O'Neill, T.W., Cockerill, W., Matthis, C., et al. (2004). Back pain, disability, and radiographic vertebral fracture in European women: a prospective study. Osteoporos Int, 15 (9): 760-5.

Onishi, J., Umegaki, H., Suzuki, Y., et al. (2004). The relationship between functional disability and depressive mood in Japanese older adult inpatients. J Ger Psych Neur, 17 (2), 93-98.

Orstavik, R.E., Haugeberg, G., Uhlig, T., et al. (2005). Incidence of vertebral deformities in 255 female rheumatoid arthritis patients measured by morphometric X-ray absorptiometry. Osteoporos Int, 16 (1): 35-42.

Oshida, Y., Ishiguro, T. (2006). Exercise therapy for the aged diabetics. Nippon Rinsho, 64 (1): 81-6.

Ostir, G.V., Markides, K.S., Black, S.A., et al. (2000). Emotional well-being predicts subsequent functional independence and survival. J Am Geriatr Soc, 48 (5): 473-8.

Otiniano, M.E., Black, S.A., Ray, L.A., et al. (2002). Correlates of diabetic complications in Mexican-American elders. Ethn Dis, 12 (2): 252-8.

Otiniano, M.E., Markides, K.S., Ottenbacher, K., et al. (2003a). Self-reported diabetic complications and 7-year mortality in Mexican American elders. Findings from a community-based study of five Southwestern states. J Diab Complic, 17 (5): 243-8.

Otiniano, M.E., Du, X., Ottenbacher, K., et al. (2003b). Lower extremity amputations in diabetic Mexican American elders: incidence, prevalence and correlate. J Diab Complic, 17 (2): 59-65.

Otiniano, M.E., Du, X.L., Ottenbacher, K., et al. (2003c). The effect of diabetes combined with stroke on disability, self-rated health, and mortality in older Mexican-Americans: results from the Hispanic EPESE. Arch Phys Med Rehabil, 84 (5): 725-30.

Ottenbacher, K.J., Ostir, G.V., Peek, M.K., et al. (2002). Diabetes mellitus as a risk factor for hip fracture in Mexican American older adults. J Gerontol A Biol Sci Med Sci, 57 (10): M648-53.

Ottenbacher, K.J., Ostir, G.V., Peek, M.K., et al. (2004). Diabetes mellitus as a risk factor for stroke incidence and mortality in Mexican American older adults. J Gerontol A Biol Sci Med Sci, 59 (6): M640-5.

Pande, I., Scott, D.L., O'Neill, T.W., et al. (2006). Quality of life, morbidity, and mortality after low trauma hip fractures in men. Ann Rheum Dis, 65 (1): 87-92.

Paquet, M., Bolduc, N., Xhignesse, M., et al. (2005). Re-engineering cardiac rehabilitation programmes: considering the patient's point of view. J Adv Nurs, 51 (6): 567-76.

Pargament, K.I. (1997). The Psychology of religion and coping: Theory, research, practice. New York: Guilford.

Park, C.L., Aldwin, C.M., Snyder, L., et al. (2005). Coping with September 11: Uncontrollable stress, PTSD, and post traumatic growth. Submitted for publication.

Parker, P.A., Baile, W.F., de Moor, C., et al. (2003). Psychosocial and demographic predictors of quality of life in a large sample of cancer patients. Psychooncology, 12 (2): 183-93.

Patankar, S.K., Larach, S.W., Ferrara, A., et al. (2003). Prospective comparison of laparoscopic vs. open resections for colorectal adenocarcinoma over a ten-year period. Dis Colon Rectum, 46, 601-611.

Patel, U.D., Young, E.W., Ojo, A.O., et al. (2005). CKD progression and mortality among older patients with diabetes. Am J Kidney Dis, 46 (3): 406-14.

PDRHealth Family Guide Series, Thomson Healthcare. (2004). Could you have "silent" diabetes? http://www.pdrhealth.com/content/life long_health/chapters/fgac24.shtml.

Pease, C.T., Bkakta, B.B., Devlin, J., et al. (1999). Does the age of onset of rheumatoid arthritis influence phenotype?: a prospective study of outcome and prognostic factors. Rheumatology, 38 (3): 228-34.

Pedro, L.W. (2001). Quality of life for long-term survivors of cancer: influencing variable. Cancer Nurs, 24 (1): 1-11.

Penning-van Beest, F.J., Goettsch, W.G., Erkens, J.A., et al. (2006). Determinants of persistence with bisphosphonates: a study in women with postmenopausal osteoporosis. Clin Ther, 28 (2): 236-42.

Penninx, B.W., van Tilburg, T., Boeke, A.J., et al. (1998). Effects of social support and personal coping resources on depressive symptoms: different for various chronic diseases? Hlth Psychol, 17 (6): 551-8.

Penninx, B.W., van Tilburg, T., Deeg, D.J., et al. (1997). Direct and buffer effects of social support and personal coping resources in individuals with arthritis. Soc Sci Med, 44 (3): 393-402.

Penttinen, J. (1995). Back pain and risk of suicide among Finnish farmers. Amer J Pub Hlth, 85 (10), 1452-1453.

Pescatello, L.S., Murphy, D., Costanzo, D. (2000). Low-intensity physical activity benefits blood lipids and lipoproteins in older adults living at home. Age Ageing, 29 (5): 433-439.

Peterson, C. (1988). Explanatory style as a risk factor for illness. Cognit Ther Res, 12, 117-130.

Pfister, A.K., Welch, C.A., Lester, M.D., et al. (2006). Cost-effectiveness strategies to treat osteoporosis in elderly women. South Med J, 99 (2): 123-31.

Philbin, E.F., McCullough, P.A., DiSalvo, T.G., et al. (2001). Underuse of invasive procedures among Medicaid patients with acute myocardial infarction. Am J Public Health, 91 (7): 1082-8.

Phillips, L. H. and Allen, R. (2004). Adult aging and the perceived intensity of emotions in faces and stories. Aging Clin Exper Res, 16, 190-199.

Pluchon, C., Simonnet, E., Toullat, G., et al. (2002). The effects of normal aging on face naming and recognition of famous people: Battery 75. Rev Neuro, 158, 703-708.

Polanczyk, C.A., Marcantonio, E., Goldman, L., et al. (2001). Impact of age on periopertive complications and length of stay in patients undergoing noncardiac surgery. Ann Intern Med, 134 (8): 637-43.

Prince, M., Harwood, R., Thomas, A. et al. (1998). A prospective population-based cohort study of the effects of disablement and social milieu on the onset and maintenance of late-life depression. Psych Med, 28, 337-350.

Prince, R.L., Devine, A., Dhaliwal, S.S., et al. (2006). Effects of calcium supplementation on clinical fracture and bone structure: results of a 5-year, double-blind, placebo-controlled trial in elderly women. Arch Intern Med, 166 (8): 869-75.

Prins, N.D., van Kijk, E.J., den Heijer, T., et al. (2005). Cerebral small-vessel disease and decline in information processing speed, executive function and memory. Brain, 128, 2034-2041.

Puett, D.W., Griffin, M.R. (1994). Published trials of nonmedicinal and noninvasive therapies for hip and knee osteoarthritis. Ann Intern Med, 121 (2): 133-40.

Puggaard, L., Larsen, J.B., Stovring, H., et al. (2000). Maximal oxygen uptake, muscle strength an walking speed in 85 year-old women: effects of increased physical activity. Aging, 12: 180-189.

Qiu, C., Winblad, B., Marengoni, A., et al. (2006). Heart failure and risk of dementia and Alzheimer disease: a population-based cohort study. Arch Intern Med, 166 (9): 1003-8.

Rabbit, P.M., Lowe, C., Scott, M., et al. (2004). Balance as a marker for global brain atrophy, blood flow and cognitive changes in old age. Unpublished manuscript.

Ragland, D.R., Santariano, W.A. and MacLeod, K.E. (2005). Driving cessation and increased depressive symptoms. Journals of Gerontology: Bio Sci Med Sci, 60, 399-403.

Raji, M.A., Tang, R.A., Heyn, P.C., et al. (2005). Screening for cognitive impairment in older adults attending an eye clinic. J Natl Med Assoc, 97 (6): 808-14.

Ramesh, H.S., Pope, D., Gennari, R., et al. (2005). Optimising surgical management of elderly cancer patients. World J Surg Oncol, 3 (1): 17.

Ranchor, A.V., Sanderman, R., Steptoe, A., et al. (2002). Pre-morbid predictors of psychological adjustment to cancer. Qual Life Res, 11 (2): 101-13.

Rankin, K.P., Baldwin, E., Pace-Savitsky, C., et al. (2005). Self awareness and personality changes in dementia. J Neuro Neurosurg Psychiatry, 76, 632-639.

Ratcliff, R., Spieler, D. and McKoon, G. (2000). Explicitly modeling the effects of aging on response time. Psychonomic Bull Rev, 7, 1-25.

Ratcliff, R., Thapar, A. and McKoon, G. (2004). A diffusion model analysis of the effects of aging on recognition memory. J Memory Language, 50, 408-424.

Rathore, S.S., Berger, A.K., Weinfurt, K.P., et al. (2000). Acute myocardial infarction complicated by atrial fibrillation in the elderly: prevalence and outcomes. Circulation, 101 (9): 969-74.

Redaelli, A., Cranor, C.W., Okano, G.J., et al. (2003). Screening, prevention and socioeconomic costs associated with the treatment of colorectal cancer. Pharmacoeconomics, 21 (17): 1213-38.

Reimer, M.A., Slaughter, S., Donaldson, C., et al. (2004). Special care facility compared with traditional environments for dementia care: a longitudinal study of quality of life. J Amer Geriatr Soc, 52: 1085.

Repetto, L. (2003). Greater risks of chemotherapy toxicity in elderly patients with cancer. J Support Oncol, 1 (4 Suppl): 18-24.

Repetto, L., Venturino, A., Fratino, L., et al. (2003). Geriatric oncology: a clinical approach to the older patient with cancer. Eur J Cancer, 39 (7): 870-80.

Retchin, S.M., Brown, R.S., Yeh, S.C., et al. (1997). Outcomes of stroke patients in Medicare fee for service and managed care. JAMA, 278 (2): 119-24.

Reuter-Lorenz, P.A. and Sylvester, C.Y. (2005). The cognitive neuroscience of working memory and aging. In R. Cabeza, L. Nyberg and D. Park (Eds.), Cognitive neuroscience of aging. New York: Oxford University Press.

Rhee, M.K., Cook, C.B., El-Kebbi, I., et al. (2005). Barriers to diabetes education in urban patients: perceptions, patterns, and associated factors. Diabetes Educ, 31 (3): 410-7.

Ribeiro, L.S., Proietti, F.A. (2004). Interrelations between fibromyalgia, thyroid autoantibodies, and depression. J Rheumatol, 31 (10): 2036-40.

Rich, M.W. (1997). Epidemiology, pathophysiology, and etiology of congestive heart failure in older adults. J Am Geriatr Soc, 45 (8): 968-74.

Rich, M.W. (2005). Heart failure in the oldest patients: the impact of comorbid conditions. Am J Geriatr Cardiol, 14 (3): 134-41.

Riegel, B.J., Dracup, K.A. (1992). Does overprotection cause cardiac invalidism after acute myocardial infarction? Heart Lung, 21 (6): 529-35.

Robbins, A.S., Rubenstein L.Z., Josephson, K.R., et al. (1989). Predictors of falls among elderly people. Results of two population-based studies. Arch Intern Med, 149: 1628-1633.

Roberts, B.W. and Delvecchio, W. F. (2000). The rank order consistency of personality traits from childhood to old age: A quantitative review of longitudinal studies. Psych Bull, 126, 3-25.

Robinson, J.D., Turner, J. (2003). Impersonal, interpersonal, and hyperpersonal social support: cancer and older adults. Health Communic, 15 (2): 227-34.

Robinson, R.L., Birnbaum, H.G., Morley, M.A., et al. (2003). Economic cost and epidemiological characteristics of patients with fibromyalgia claims. J Rheumatol 30 (6): 1318-25.

Robison, J., Curry, L., Gruman, C., et al. (2003). Depression in later-life Puerto Rican primary care patients: the role of illness, stress, social integration and religiosity. Int Psychoger, 15 (3), 239-251.

Roche, R.J., Forman, W.B., Rhyne, R.L. (1997). Formal geriatric assessment, An imperative for the older person with cancer. Cancer Pract, 5 (2): 81-6.

Rodriguez, K.L., Young, A.J. (2006). Patients' and healthcare providers' understanding of life-sustaining treatment: are perceptions of goals shared or divergent? Soc Sci Med, 62 (1): 125-33.

Roman, M.J., Moeller, E., Davis, A., et al. (2006). Preclinical carotid atherosclerosis in patients with rheumatoid arthritis. Ann Intern Med, 144 (4): 249-56.

Romanelli, J., Fauerbach, J.A., Bush, D.E., et al. (2002). The significance of depression in older patients after myocardial infarction. J Am Geriatr Soc, 50 (5): 817-22.

Roscoe, L.A., Malphurs, J.E., Dragovic, L.J., et al. (2003). Antecedents of euthanasia and suicide among older women. J Amer Med Womens Assoc, 58 (1), 44-48.

Rosenstock, J. (2001). Management of type 2 diabetes mellitus in the elderly: special considerations. Drugs Aging, 18 (1): 31-44.

Rossi, A., Colantuoni, G., Maione, P., et al. (2005). Chemotherapy of breast cancer in the elderly. Curr Med Chem, 12 (3): 297-310.

Roumie, C.L., Griffin, M.R. (2004). Over-the-counter analgesics in older adults: a call for improved labeling and consumer education. Drugs Aging, 21 (8): 485-98.

Rowe, J.W., Kahn, R.L. (1997). Successful aging. The Gerontologist, 37: 433-440.

Ruo, B., Rumsfeld, J.S., Hlatky, M.A., et al. (2003). Depressive symptoms and health-related quality of life: the Heart and Soul Study. JAMA, 290 (2): 215-21.

Rustoen, T., Wahl, A.K., Hanestad, B.R., et al. (2005). Age and the experience of chronic pain: differences in health and quality of life among younger, middle-aged, and older adults. Clin J Pain, 21 (6): 513-23.

Ruthman, J.L., Ferrans, C.E. (2004). Efficacy of a video for teaching patients about prostate cancer screening and treatment. Am J Health Promot, 18 (4): 292-5.

Ryan, A.S., Hurlbut, D.E., Lott, M.E., et al. (2001). Insulin action after resistive training in insulin resistant older men and women. J Am Geriatr Soc, 49(3): 247-253.

Sabel, M.S., Strecher, V.J., Schwartz, J.L., et al. (2005). Patterns of Internet use and impact on patients with melanoma. J Am Acad Dermatol 52 (5): 779-85.

Sale, J.E., Gignac, M., Hawker, G. (2006). How "bad" does the pain have to be? A qualitative study examining adherence to pain medication in older adults with osteoarthritis. Arthritis Rheum, 55 (2): 272-8.

Salthouse, T.A. (1985). Speed of behavior and its implications for cognition. In J.E. Birren and K.W. Schaie (Eds), Handbook of the psychology of aging (2nd edition). New York: Van Norstrand Reinhold.

Salthouse, T.A. (1998). Relation of successive percentiles of reaction time distributions to cognitive variables and adult age. Intelligence, 26, 153-166.

Salthouse, T.A. and Caja, S.J. (2000). Structural constraints on process explanations in cognitive aging. Psych Aging, 15, 44-55.

Salthouse, T.A. (2001). Structural models of the relations between age and measures of cognitive functioning. Intelligence, 29, 93-115.

Salthouse, T.A. and Ferrer-Caja, E. (2003). What needs to be explained to account for age-related effects on multiple cognitive variables? Psych Aging, 18, 91-110.

Samuel-Hodge, C.D., Skelly, A.H., Headen, S., et al. (2005). Familial roles of older African-American women with type 2 diabetes: testing of a new multiple care-giving measure. Ethn Dis, 15 (3): 436-43.

Sanchez Perales, M.C., Garcia Cortes, M.J., Borrego Utiel, F.J., et al. (2005). Incidence and risk factors for non-traumatic lower extremity amputation in hemodialysis patients. Nefrologia, 25 (4): 399-406.

Sandstrom, M.J., Keefe, F.J. (1998). Self-management of fibromyalgia: the role of formal coping skills training and physical exercise training programs. Arthritis Care Res, 11 (6): 432-47.

Santini, F., Montalbanao, G., Messina, A., et al. (2006). Survival and quality of life afterrepair of acute type A aortic dissection in patients aged 75 years and older justify intervention. Eur J Cardiothorac Surg, 29 (3): 386-91.

Saykin, A.J., Wishart, H.A., Rabin, L.A., et al. (2006). Older adults with cognitive complaints show brain atrophy similar to that of annestic MCI. Neurology, 67, 834-842.

Schiel, R., Braun, A., Muller, R., et al. (2004). A structured treatment and educational program for patients with type 2 diabetes mellitus, insulin therapy and impaired cognitive function (DiKol). Med Klin (Munich) 99 (6); 285-92.

Schiel, R., Ulbrich, S., Muller, U.A. (1998). Quality of diabetes care, diabetes knowledge and risk of severe hypoglycaemia one and four years after participation in a 5-day structured treatment and teaching pro-gramme for intensified insulin therapy. Diab Metab, 24 (6): 509-14.

Schiff, M.H., Yu, E.B., Weinblatt, M.E., et al. (2006). Long-term experi-ence with etanercept in the treatment of rheumatoid arthritis in elderly and younger patients: patient-reported outcomes from multiple con-trolled and open-label extension studies. Drugs Aging, 23 (2): 167-78.

Schneider, B.A., Daneman, M. and Murphy, D.R. (2005). Speech compre-hension difficulties in older adults: cognitive slowing or age-related changes in hearing? Psych Aging, 20, 261-271.

Schneider, R.H., Alexander, C.N., Staggers, F., et al. (2005). Long-term effects of stress reduction on mortality in persons > or = 55 years of age with systemic hypertension. Am J Cardiol, 95 (9): 1060-4.

Schneider, S., Schmitt, G., Mau, H., et al. (2005). Prevalence and corre-lates of osteoarthritis in Germany. Representative data from the First National Health Survey. Orthopade, 34 (8): 782-90.

Schneiderman, N., Antoni, M.H., Saab, P.G., et al. (2001). Psychosocial and biobehavioral aspects of chronic disease management. Ann Rev Psych, 52, 555-580.

Schoenberg, N.E., Amey, C.H., Coward, R.T. (1998). Stories of meaning: lay perspectives on the origin and management of noninsulin depend-ent diabetes mellitus among older women in the United States. Soc Sci Med, 47 (12): 2113-25.

Schoenberg, N.E., Drew, E.M., Stoller, E.P., et al. (2005). Situating stress: les-sons from lay discourses on diabetes. Med Anthropol Q, 19 (2): 71-93.

Schoenberg, N.E., Drungle, S.C. (2001). Barriers to non-insulin dependent diabetes mellitus (NIDDM) self-care practices among older women. J Aging Health, 13 (4): 443-66.

Schofield, P., Ball, D., Smith, J.D., et al. (2004). Optimism and survival in lung carcinoma patients. Cancer, 100, 1276-1282.

Schulz, R., Bookwala, J., Knapp, J.E., et al. (1996). Pessimism, age and cancer mortality. Psychology and Aging, 11, 304-309.

Schwartz, A.V., Sellmeyer, D.E., Ensrud, K.E., et al. (2001). Older women with diabetes have increased risk of fracture: A prospective study. J Clin Endocrinol Metab, 86: 32-38.

Schwartz, A.V., Sellmeyer, D.E., Strotmeyer, E.S., et al. (2005). Diabetes and bone loss at the hip in older black and white adults. J Bone Miner Res, 20 (4): 596-603.

Schwarz, K.A., Elman, C.S. (2003). Identification of factors predictive of hospital readmissions for patients with heart failure. Heart Lung, 32 (2): 88-99.

Seeman, E. (2006). Strontium ranelate: vertebral and non-vertebral fracture risk reduction. Curr Opin Rheumatol, 18 Suppl 1: S17-20.

Segestrom, S.C. (2001). Optimism, goal conflict and stressor-related immune change. J Behav Med, 24 (5), 441-467.

Setter, S.M., Corbett, C.F., Higgins, T.C., et al. (2005). Effectiveness of an osteoporosis intervention among older adults residing in assisted living facilities. Consult Pharm, 20 (5): 416-23.

Sewell, K.L. (1998). Rheumatoid arthritis in older adults. Clin Geriatr Med, 14 (3): 475-94.

Sherwood, P., Given, B.A., Given, C.W., et al. (2005). A cognitive behavioral intervention for symptom management in patients with advanced cancer. Oncol Nurs Forum, 32 (6): 1190-8.

Shi, L., Singh, D.A. (2004). Delivering health care in America. A systems approach. Sudbury, MA: Jones and Bartlett Publishers.

Shibata, H. (2001). Nutritional factors on longevity and quality of life in Japan. J Nutrition Hlth Aging, 5: 97-102.

Shih, M., Hootman, J.M., Kruger, J., et al. (2006). Physical activity in men and women with arthritis: National Health Interview Survey, 2002. Am J Prev Med, 30 (5): 385-93.

Shneker, B.F., McAuley, J.W. (2005). Pregabalin: a new neuromodulator with broad therapeutic indications. Ann Pharmacother, 39 (12): 2029-37.

Silver, M.A., Peacock, W.F., 4th, et al. (2006). Optimizing treatment and outcomes in acute heart failure: beyond initial triage. Congest Heart Fail, 12 (3): 137-45.

Silverman, S.L., Piziak, V.K., Chen, P., et al. (2005). Relationship of health related quality of life to prevalent and new or worsening back pain in postmenopausal women with osteoporosis. J Rheumatol, 32 (12): 2405-9.

Simon, S.R., Chan, K.A., Soumerai, S.B., et al. (2005). Potentially inappropriate medication use by elderly persons in U.S. Health Maintenance Organizations, 2000-2001. J Am Geriatr Soc, 53 (2): 227-32.

Simon, S.R., Smith, D.H., Feldstein, A.C., et al. (2006). Computerized prescribing alerts and group academic detailing to reduce the use of potentially inappropriate medications in older people. J Am Geriatr Soc, 54 (6): 963-8.

Sinclair, A.J., Bayer, A.J., Girling, A.J., et al. (2000). Older adults, diabetes mellitus and visual acuity: a community-based case-control study. Age Ageing, 29 (4): 335-9.

Sinclair, A.J., Conroy, S.P., Davies, M., et al. (2005). Post-discharge home-based support for older cardiac patients: a randomised controlled trial. Age Ageing, 34 (4): 338-43.

Sinclair, A.J., Girling, A.J., Bayer, A.J. (2000). Cognitive dysfunction in older subjects with diabetes mellitus: impact on diabetes self-management and use of care services. All Wales Research into Elderly (AWARE) Study. Diabetes Res Clin Pract, 50 (3): 203-12.

Sleath, B., Rubin, R.H., Campbell, W, et al. (2001). Ethnicity and physician-older patient communication about alternative therapies. J Altern Complement Med, 7 (4): 329-35.

Small, B.J. and Backman, L. (1997). Cognitive correlates of mortality: Evidence from a population-based sample of very old adults. Psych Aging, 12, 309-313.

Small, B.J., Hertzog, C., Hultsch, D.F., et al. (2003). Stability and change in adult personality over 6 years: Findings from the Victoria longitudinal study. J Ger: Psych Sci Soc Sci, 58B, 166-176.

Smalley, W.E., Griffin, M.R., Fought, R.L., et al. (1996). Excess costs from gastrointestinal disease associated with nonsteroidal anti-inflammatory drugs. J Gen Intern Med, 11 (8): 461-9.

Smith, M.T., Perlis, M.L. and Haythornthwaite, J.A. (2004). Suicidal ideation in outpatients with chronic musculoskeletal pain: an exploratory study of the role of sleep onset insomnia and pain intensity. Clin J Pain, 20 (2), 111-118.

Smith, N.L., Savage, P.J., Heckbert, S.R., et al. (2002). Glucose, blood pressure, and lipid control in older people with and without diabetes mellitus: the Cardiovascular Health Study. J Am Geriatr Soc, 50 (3): 416-23.

Smith, T.W. and Spiro, A., III (2002). Personality, health and aging: Prolegomenon for the next generation, J Res Per, 36, 363-394.

Smitz, S. (2005). The care of the older person with diabetes mellitus. Rev Med Liege, 60 (5-6): 433-8.

Solomon, D.H., Avorn, J., Katz, J.N., et al. (2005). Compliance with osteoporosis medications. Arch Intern Med, 165 (20): 2414-9.

Sotile, W.M., Miller, H.S. (1998). Helping older patients cope with cardiac and pulmonary disease. J Cardiopulm Rehabil, 18 (2): 124-8.

Soumerai, S.B., McLaughlin, T.J., Gurwitz, J.H., et al. (1999). Timeliness and quality of care for elderly patients with acute myocardial infarction under health maintenance organization vs. fee-for-service insurance. Arch Intern Med, 159 (17): 2013-20.

Spencer, W.D. and Raz, N. (1995). Differential effects of aging on memory for content and context: a meta-analysis. Psych Aging, 10, 527-539.

Speziale, G., Bonifazi, R., Cavagnaro, P., et al. (2005). Cardiac surgery in octogenarians: a six-year follow-up with a multidimensional intervention. Ital Heart J Suppl, 6 (10): 674-81.

Squiers, L., Finney Rutten, L.J., Treiman, K., et al. (2005). Cancer patients' information needs across the cancer continuum: evidence from the cancer information service. J Health Commun, 10 (Suppl 1): 15-34.

Stack, A.G., Messana, J.M. (2000). Renal replacement therapy in the elderly: medical, ethical, and psychosocial considerations. Adv Ren Replace Ther, 7 (1): 52-62.

Stang, P.E., Brandenburg, N.A., Lane, M.C., et al. (2006). Mental and physical comorbid conditions and days in role among persons with arthritis. Psychosom Med, 68 (1): 152-8.

Starr, J.M., McGurn, B., Whiteman, M., et al. (2004). Life long changes in cognitive ability are associated with prescribed medications in old age. Int J Ger Psychiatry, 19, 327-332.

Stein, C.M., Griffin, M.R., Taylor, J.A., et al. (2001). Educational program for nursing home physicians and staff to reduce use of non-steroidal anti-inflammatory drugs among nursing home residents. Med Care, 39 (5): 436-45.

Stenager, E.N., Stenager, E. and Jensen, K. (1994). Attempted suicide, depression and physical diseases: a 1-year follow-up study. Psychotherapy Psychosom, 61 (1-2), 65-73.

Stern, R.A., Davis, J.D., Rogers, B.L., et al. (2004). Preliminary study of the relationship between thyroid status and cognitive and neuropsychiatric functioning in euthyroid patients with Alzheimer dementia. Cognitive Behav Neuro, 17, 219-223.

Stern, Y., Hlabeck, C., Moeller, J., et al. (2005). Brain networks associated with cognitive reserve in healthy young and old adults. Cerebral Cortex, 15, 394-402.

Stevenson, J.S. (2005). Alcohol use, misuse, abuse and dependence in later adulthood. Ann Rev Nurs Res, 23, 245-280.

Strandberg, T.E., Strandberg, A., Rantanen, K., et al. (2004). Low cholesterol, mortality and quality of life in old age during a 39-year follow-up. J Amer Coll Cardiol, 44: 1002-1008.

Strawbridge, W.J., Deleger, S., Roberts, R.E., et al. (2002). Physical activity reduces the risk of subsequent depression for older adults. Amer J Epi, 156 (4), 328-334.

Strawbridge, W.J., Wallhagen, M.I. and Cohen, R.D. (2002). Successful aging and well-being. The Gerontologist, 42: 727-733.

Sturnieks, D.L., Tiedemann, A., Chapman, K., et al. (2004). Physiological risk factors for falls in older people with lower limb arthritis. J Rheumatol, 31 (11): 2272-9.

Sullivan, M.J., Reesor, K., Mikail, S., et al. (1992). The treatment of depression in chronic low back pain: review and recommendations. Pain, 50, 5-13.

Surtees, P., Wainwright, N., Luben, R., et al. (2003). Sense of coherence and mortality in men and women in the EPIC-Norfolk United Kingdom prospective cohort study, Amer J Epidemiol, 158, 1202-1209.

Tagliareni, E., et al. (1991). Participatory clinical education. Nurs Hlth Care, 12 (5): 248.

Tak, S.H. (2006). An insider perspective of daily stress and coping in elders with arthritis. Orthop Nurs, 25 (2): 127-32.

Tak, S.H., Laffrey, S.C. (2003). Life satisfaction and its correlates in older women with osteoarthritis. Orthop Nurs, 22 (3). 182-9.

T'ang, J., Chan, C., Chan, N.F., et al. (1999). A survey of elderly diabetic patients attending a community clinic in Hong Kong. Patient Educ Couns, 36 (3): 259-70.

Tanko, L.B., Christiansen, C., Cox, D.A., et al. (2005). Relationship between osteoporosis and cardiovascular disease in postmenopausal women. J Bone Miner Res 20 (11): 1912-20.

Taylor-Piliae, R.E., Haskell, W.L., Waters, C.M., et al. (2006). Change in perceived psychosocial status following a 12-week Tai Chi exercise programme. J Adv Nurs, 54 (3): 313-29.

Tekkis, P.P., Poloniecki, J.D., Thompson, M.R., et al. (2002a) ACPGBI Colorectal Cancer Study 2002—Part A: unadjusted outcomes.

Tekkis, P.P., Poloniecki, J.D., Thompson, M.R., et al. (2002b) ACPGBI Colorectal Cancer Study 2002—Part B: risk adjusted outcomes The ACPGBI Colorectal Cancer Model.

Tennant, C. and McLean, L. (2001). The impact of emotions on coronary heart disease risk, J Cardiov Risk, 8, 175-183.

Terrell, K.M., Heard, K., Miller, D.K. (2006). Prescribing to older ED patients. Am J Emerg Med, 24 (4): 468-78.

Thearle, M., Brillantes, A.M. (2005). Unique characteristics of the geriatric diabetic population and the role for therapeutic strategies than enhance glucagon-like peptide-1 activity. Curr Opin Clin Nutr Metab Care, 8 (11): 9-16.

Thewes, B., Butow, P., Girgis, A., et al. (2004). The psychosocial needs of breast cancer survivors; a qualitative study of the shared and unique needs of younger versus older survivors. Psychooncology, 13 (3): 177-89.

Thomas, P., Hazif-Thomas, C., Saccardy, F., et al. (2004). Loss of motivation and frontal dysfunction. Role of the white matter change. Encephale, 30, 52-59.

Thoresen, C.E., Harris, A.H. and Luskin, F. (2000). Forgiveness and health: An unanswered question. In M.E. McCullough, K.I. Pargament and C.E. Thoresen (Eds.), Forgiveness: Theory, research and practice. New York: Guilford.

Tinetti, M.E., Williams, T.F., Mayewski, R. (1986). Fall risk index for elderly patients based on number of chronic disabilities. Am J Med, 80: 429-434.

Torras-Garcia, M., Costa-Miserachs, D., Coll-Andreu, M., et al. (2005). Decreased anxiety levels related to aging. Exper Brain Res, 164 (2), 177-184.

Travis, S.S., Buchanan, R.J., Wang, S., et al. (2004). Analyses of nursing home residents with diabetes at admission. J Am Med Dir Assoc, 5 (5): 320-7.

Treharne, G.J., Hale, E.D., Lyons, A.C., et al. (2005). Cardiovascular disease and psychological morbidity among rheumatoid arthritis patients. Rheumatology (Oxford), 44 (2): 241-6.

Trief, P.M., Grant, W., Elbert, K., et al. (1998). Family environment, glycemic control, and the psychosocial adaptation of adults with diabetes. Diabetes Care, 21 (2): 241-5.

Tsai, P.F., Tak, S., Moore, C., et al. (2003). Testing a theory of chronic pain. J Adv Nurs, 43(2): 158-69.

Tsuji, T., Matsuyama, Y., Sato, K., et al. (2001). Epidemiology of low back pain in the elderly: correlation with lumbar lordosis. J Orthop Sci, 6 (4): 307-11.

Tun, P.A., Perlmuter, L.C., Russo, P., et al. (1987). Memory self-assessment and performance in aged diabetics and non-diabetics. Exp Aging Res, 13 (3): 151-7.

Turesson, C., O'Fallon, W.M., Crowson, C.S., et al. (2002). Occurrence of extraarticular disease manifestations is associated with excess mortality in a community based cohort of patient with rheumatoid arthritis. J Rheumatol, 29 (1): 62-7.

Ubel, P.A. (2001). Physicians, thou shall ration: the necessary role of bedside rationing: the necessary role of bedside rationing in controlling healthcare cost. Healthc Pap, 2 (2): 10-21.

Ueda, T., Tamaki, M., Kageyama, S., et al. (2000). Urinary incontinence among community-dwelling people aged 40 years or older in Japan. Prevalence, risk factors, knowledge and self-perception. Int J Urol, 7: 95-103.

USDHHS (2002). Health, United States, 2005. National Center for Health Statistics.

USDHHS (2005). Health, United States, 2005. National Center for Health Statistics.

U.S. Food and Drug Administration (1996). Growing older, eating better. FDA Consumer Magazine, March issue, Pub No. FDA 04-1301C.

U.S. Surgeon General (1990). Health benefits of quitting smoking. USDHHS, CDC.http://profiles.nlm.nih.gov/NN/B/B/C/T_/nnbbct.pdf.

University of Manchester (2005). Brightly coloured fruit and vegetable may protect against arthritis. http://www.emaxhealth.com/97/3178.html.

Unutzer, J., Patrick, D., Marmon, T., et al. (2002). Depressive symptoms and mortality in a prospective study of 2,558 older adults. Amer J Ger Psych, 10 (5): 521-30.

Vailas, L.I., Nitzke, S.A., Becker, M., et al. (1998). Risk indictors for malnutrition are associated inversely with quality of life for participants in meal programs for older adults. J Amer Diet Assoc, 98, 548-553.

Valentijn, S.A., van Boxel, M.P., van Hooren, S.A., et al. (2005). Change in sensory functioning predicts change in cognitive functioning: results from a 6-year follow-up in the Maastricht aging study. J Amer Ger Society, 53, 374-380.

Valmadrid, C.T., Klein, R., Moss, S.E., et al. (2000). The risk of cardiovascular disease mortality associated with microalbuminuria and gross proteinuria in persons with older-onset diabetes mellitus. Arch Intern Med, 160 (8): 1093-100.

Van Gool, C.H., Kempen, G.I., Pennis, B.W., et al. (2005). Impact of depression on disablement in late middle aged and older persons: results from the Longitudinal Aging Study Amsterdam. Soc Sci Med, 60 (1), 25-36.

Verbrugge, L.M., Juarez, L. (2006). Profile of arthritis disability: II. Arthritis Rheum, 55 (1): 102-13.

Verhaegen, P. and Salthouse, T.A. (1997). Meta-analyses of age-cognition relations in adulthood: estimates of linear and non-linear age effects and structural models. Psych Bull, 122, 231-249.

Vigorito, C., Incalzi, R.A., Acanfora, D., et al. (2003). Recommendations for cardiovascular rehabilitation in the very elderly. Monaldi Arch Chest Dis, 60 (1): 25-39.

Vinik, A.I. (1999). Diabetic neuropathy. Pathogenesis and therapy. Am J Med, 107, 17S-26S.

Vitaliano, P.P., Russo, J. and Niauraa, R. (1995). Plasmid lipids and their relationships with psychosocial factors in older adults. J Ger: Series B: Psycholog Sci Soc Sci, 50, P18-P24.

Volk, R.J., Spann, S.J., Cass, A.R., et al. (2003). Patient education for informed decision making about prostate cancer screening: a randomized controlled trial with 1-year follow-up. Ann Fam Med, 1 (1): 22-8.

Volpato, S., Pahor, M., Ferrucci, L., et al. (2004). Relationship of alcohol intake with inflammatory markers and plasminogen activator inhibitor-1 in well-functioning older adults: the Health, Aging, and Body Composition study. Circulation, 109 (5): 607-12.

Von Goeler, D.S., Rosal, M.C., Ockene, J.K., et al. (2003). Self-management of type 2 diabetes: a survey of low-income urban Puerto Ricans. Diab Educ, 29 (4): 663-72.

Von Moltke, L.L., Greenblatt, D.J., Harmatz, J.S., et al. (2000). Psychotropic drug metabolism in old age: principles and problems of assessment. http://www.acnp.org/g4GN401000140/CH137.html.

Wachtel, M.S. (2005). Family poverty accounts for differences in lower-extremity amputation rates of minorities 50 years old or more with diabetes. J Natl Med Assoc, 97 (3): 334-8.

Wanebo, H.J., Cole, B., Chung, M., et al. (1997). Is surgical management compromised in elderly patients with breast cancer? Ann Surg, 225 (5): 579-86; discussion 586-9.

Ware, J.E., Jr., Bayliss, M.S., Rogers, W.H., et al. (1996). Differences in 4-year health outcomes for elderly and poor, chronically ill patients treated in HMO and fee-for-service systems. Results from the Medical Outcomes Study. JAMA, 276 (13): 1039-47.

Weaver Cargin, J., Maruff, P., Collie, A., et al. (2006). Mild memory impairment in healthy older adults is distinct from normal aging. Brain Cognition, 60, 146-155.

Webb, R., Brammah, T., Lunt, M., et al. (2003). Prevalence and predictors of intense, chronic, and disabling neck and back pain in the UK general population. Spine, 28 (11): 1195-202.

Weiner, D.K., Kim, Y.S., Bonino, P., et al. (2006). Low back pain in older adults: are we utilizing healthcare resources wisely? Pain Med, 7 (2): 143-50.

Wen, L.K., Shepherd, M.D., Parchman, M.L. (2004). Family support, diet, and exercise among older Mexican Americans with type 2 diabetes. Diabetes Educ, 30 (6): 980-93.

Wengstrom, Y., Haggmark, C., Forsberg, C. (2001). Coping with radiation therapy: effects of a nursing intervention on coping ability for women with breast cancer. Int J Nurs Pract, 7 (1): 8-15.

West, C., McDowell, J. (2002). The distress experienced by people with type 2 diabetes. Br J Community Nurs, 7 (12): 606-13.

Weycker, D., Yu, E.B., Wooley, J.M., et al. (2005). Retrospective study of the costs of care during the first year of therapy with etanercept or infliximab among patients > or = 65 years with rheumatoid arthritis. Clint Ther, 27 (5): 646-56.

Wheeler, J.R., Janz, N.K., Dodge, J.A. (2003). Can a disease self-management program reduce health care costs? The case of older women with heart disease. Med Care, 41 (6): 706-15.

White, J.V. (2002). Diabetes mellitus. Nutrition management for older adults. Washington, D.C.: Nutrition Screening Initiative (NSI). 14 pages.

White, K.P., Speechley, M., Harth, M. (1999). The London Fibromyalgia Epidemiology Study: comparing the demographic and clinical characteristics in 100 random community cases of fibromyalgia versus controls. J Rheumatol, 26 (7): 1577-85.

White House Conference on Aging (2005), San Diego, CA.

Wiggins, R.D. (2004). Quality of life in the third age: key predictors of the CADP-19 measure. Aging Soc, 24: 693-708.

Wilkins, C.H., Birge, S.J. (2005). Prevention of osteoporotic fractures in the elderly. Am J Med, 118 (11): 1190-5.

Williams, J.W., Jr., Katon, W., Lin, E.H., et al. (2004). The effectiveness of depression care management on diabetes-related outcomes in older patients. Ann Intern Med, 140 (12): 1015-24.

Williams, R.B. (2000). Psychological factors, health and disease: The impact of aging and the life cycle. In S.B. Manuck, R. Jennings, B.S. Rabin and A. Baum (Eds.), Behavior, health and aging, (pp. 135-151). Mahwah, N.J.: Lawrence Erlbaum.

Williams, S.A., Schreier, A.M. (2005). The role of education in managing fatigue, anxiety, and sleep disorders in women undergoing chemotherapy for breast cancer. Appl Nurs Res, 18 (3): 138-47.

Wilson, R.S., Krueger, K.R., Arnold, S.E., et al. (2006). Childhood adversity and psychosocial adjustment in old age. Amer J Ger Psych, 14 (4), 307-315.

Wilson, R.S., Mendes de Leon, C.F., Bienas, J.L., et al. (2004). Personality and mortality in old age. J Ger: Psychol Sci, 59B, 110-116.

Wirth, M.P., Froehner, M. (2000). Co-morbidity in prostate cancer. Aging Male, 3 (3): 132-136.

Wolfe, F., Ross, K., Anderson, J., et al. (1995). The prevalence and characteristics of fibromyalgia in the general population. Arthritis Rheum, 38 (1): 19-28.

Wolff, J.L., et al. (2002). Prevalence, expenditures, and complications of multiple chronic conditions in the elderly. Arch Int Med, 162 (20): 2269-2276.

Worthington, E.L. (2004). Commentary: Unforgiveness, forgiveness, religion and health during aging. In K.W. Schaie, N. Krause and A. Booth (Eds.), Religious influences on health and well-being among the elderly. New York: Springer.

Wray, L.A., Ofstedal, M.B., Langa, K.M., et al. (2005). The effect of diabetes on disability in middle-aged and older adults. J Gerontol A Biol Sci Med Sci, 60 (9): 1206-11.

Wright, J.G., Coyte, P., Hawker, G., et al. (1995). Variation in orthopedic surgeons' perceptions of the indications for and outcomes of knee replacement. Can Med Assoc J, 152 (5): 687-97.

Wu, J.H., Haan, M.N., Liang, J., et al. (2003). Diabetes as a predictor of change in functional status among older Mexican-Americans: a population-based cohort study. Diab Care, 26 (2): 314-9.

Yamamoto, H. and Shimada, H. (2006). Cognitive aging mechanism of signaling effects on the memory for procedural sentences. Shinrigaku Kenkyu, 77, 278-284.

Yang, Y. and George, L.K. (2005). Functional disability, disability transitions and depressive symptoms in late life. J Aging Hlth, 17 (3), 263-292.

Yepes-Rios, M., Reimann, J.O., Talavera, A.C., et al. (2006). Colorectal cancer screening among Mexican Americans at a community clinic. Am J Prev Med, 30 (3): 204-10.

Zacks, R.T., Hasher, L. and Li, K.Z.H. (2000). Human memory. In F.I.M. Craik and T.A. Salthouse (Eds), Handbook of aging and cognition (2nd edition). Mahwah, NJ: Erlbaum.

Zareba, G. (2005). Pregabalin: a new agent for the treatment of neuropathic pain. Drugs Today (Barc), 41 (8): 509-16.

Zelinski, E. M. and Burnight, K. P. (1997). Sixteen year longitudinal and time lag changes in memory and cognition in older adults. Psych Aging, 12, 503-513.

Zeyfang, A. (2005). Structured educational programs for geriatric patients with diabetes mellitus. MMW Fortschr Med, 147 (26): 43, 45-6.

About the Authors

Dr. Stephen J. Morewitz is President of the consulting firm, STEPHEN J. MOREWITZ, Ph.D., & ASSOCIATES, Buffalo Grove, IL and San Francisco and Tarzana, CA, which was founded in 1988. He is Adjunct Professor and Past Research Dean at the California School of Podiatric Medicine at Samuel Merritt College, Oakland, CA, and a Lecturer in the Graduate Health Care Administration Program, Department of Public Affairs and Administration, California State University, East Bay. He has been on the faculty or staffs of Michael Reese Hospital, University of Illinois at Chicago, College of Medicine and School of Public Health, DePaul University, and Argonne National Laboratory, Division of Biological and Medical Research. Dr. Morewitz is the author of more than 80 publications, including *Chronic Diseases and Health Care: New Trends in Diabetes, Arthritis, Fibromyalgia, Osteoporosis, Back Pain, Cardiovascular Disease and Cancer* (New York: Springer, 2006) and the award-winning book, *Domestic Violence and Maternal and Child Health* (New York: Springer, 2004).

Dr. Mark L. Goldstein, Ph.D., is a licensed clinical psychologist in Illinois. Dr. Goldstein has a private practice specializing in forensic psychology and counseling. He is also an adjunct professor at the Chicago School of Professional Psychology and consultant to a suburban school system. Dr. Goldstein received his Ph.D. from the University of Florida and was previously a core faculty member at the Illinois School of Professional Psychology and adjunct professor at the University of Illinois College of Medicine and Roosevelt University. He is the editor of a book, *Innovations in Behavioral Science Education*, and the author of numerous professional articles.

Author Index

Subject Index